Nursing Management
of the Patient with Pain

Nursing Management of the Patient with Pain

MARGO McCAFFERY R.N., M.S.

Formerly Assistant Professor of
Pediatric Nursing
University of California, Los Angeles

J. B. LIPPINCOTT COMPANY
Philadelphia • Toronto

Distributed in Great Britain by
Blackwell Scientific Publications
Oxford, London and Edinburgh

ISBN-0-397-54121-X

Library of Congress Catalog Card Number 70-37295

Printed in the United States of America

Library of Congress Cataloging in Publication Data

McCaffery, Margo
    Nursing management of the patient with pain.

    Bibliography: p.
    1. Nurse and patient. 2. Pain. I. Title
RT86.M22   610.73   70-37295
ISBN 0-397-54121-X

    3   4   2

TO MY HUSBAND BOB

who helped me to tolerate pain
and then made it possible for
me to write this book.

Preface

The purpose of the book is to help the nurse to bring some measure of relief and comfort to the patient who experiences pain. Of all the members of the health team, it is she who is in a position to have the most constant contact with the patient with pain. The nurse has a unique contribution to make in his care. In this book an attempt is made to identify precisely what that contribution may be.

Pain remains a complex, mysterious phenomenon. It cannot be completely or simply understood. Hence, a wide variety of sociological, psychological and physiological concepts covered herein provide the basis for furnishing the nursing practitioner and student with a rational approach to the care of the patient with pain. Research studies, theories and principles are combined with specific suggestions and clinical examples of ways in which nurses may utilize this knowledge in everyday practice.

The content is not limited to any particular clinical setting or type of patient. The care of the patient with pain is approached by identifying principles and applying them to nursing care. Principles are applied to the care of children and adults in a variety of clinical settings, including outpatient clinics and hospital units such as maternity, medicine and surgery.

To facilitate the application of knowledge and understanding to nursing practice, content is presented in a problem-solving framework. A chapter is devoted to each element of the problem-solving process. Scientific knowledge and clinical application are discussed in terms of their relevance to each problem-solving element. The chapters and discussions proceed logically, in a step-by-step fashion through nursing assessment, nursing diagnosis, nursing intervention and evaluation of nursing intervention. Using this problem-solving framework, all content is presented within the context of what is useful in actual nursing care. The framework also lends itself well to the incorporation of forthcoming knowledge about the care of the patient with pain.

A section titled "Further Exploration" will appear at the end of each chapter for the purpose of raising questions about the material in that chapter. These questions may include possible disagreements with the author's beliefs and approaches, sources of additional information, arguments against theories and research findings, or suggestions for further research, particularly nursing research. Such questions are usually either quite speculative, mostly a matter of opinion, or simply unanswered questions. They are not mentioned within the body of the chapter because they might tend to distract from the practical application of knowledge to patient care.

The patient experiencing pain is viewed as a total, integrated person with a variety of physical, emotional and intellectual needs and experiences, all of which influence his pain experience. Pain is merely a portion of the patient's life that is abstracted for analysis. Pain relief is acheived only by retaining the concept of the total person. The suggested nursing activities for pain relief include the assessment and management of the many facets of the patient. The nurse is seen as collaborating with the individual patient in acheiving the goal of pain relief.

It is hoped that this book will contribute not only to the care of the patient with pain but also to the care of patients with other problems. The demonstration of the application of scientific theory to nursing practice may enhance the nurse's ability to bridge the gap between other theory and nursing practice, assisting her to make her own applications of theory from the ever-increasing body of scientific knowledge. The fact that principles are applied to many types of patients may be particularly helpful to the student who is learning to transfer knowledge from one situation to another. The discussion and application of a variety of concepts such as powerlessness, cognitive dissonance and sensory restriction may serve as a means of introducing the student to new ideas that later can be elaborated upon as separate topics or in relation to other patient problems. Many of the intervention methods such as individual patient-teaching, teaching a group of patients and behavior therapy are equally applicable to patients other than those experiencing pain. In addition, the adherence to a problem-solving process may assist the nurse in using this logical approach in the care of all patients. Finally, the emphasis on involving the patient in plans for providing pain relief may help the nurse to gain a greater appreciation of the necessity of seeing the patient as a total human being and of attempting to maintain his integrity by working with him to achieve individualized goals.

Acknowledgements

The people to/whom I am most indebted are the patients who shared with me their painful experiences and the students who over the years shared with me their clinical experiences and asked me hundreds of relevant and probing questions about how to help the patient with pain.

I also wish to express my deepest appreciation to Miss Noreen Meinhart who carefully reviewed the major portion of the manuscript. I am also grateful to Mrs. Doris Holm, Mrs. Karen Kay and Mrs. Sharon Reeder for their comments on certain parts of the manuscript and to Mrs. Nancy English for her assistance with reviewing the literature.

Some recognition is due my daughter Melissa who spent the first year of her life surrounded with papers, journals, books and a typewriter. Without her dependable long and daily naps it would have taken much longer to write this book.

Contents

The Mystery of Pain

Pain has an element of blank:
It cannot recollect
When it begun, or if there were
A day when it was not.

It has no future but itself,
Its infinite realms contain
Its past, enlightened to perceive
New periods of pain.

Emily Dickinson

Chapter 1

Pain in the Context of Nursing Care

Pain is one of the universal human experiences—expressions of pain know no language barrier. Yet pain defies satisfactory definition. In many ways pain remains a mystery. Through the ages pain has been a subject of inquiry for almost every professional discipline—philosophy, theology, medicine, sociology, psychology, physiology, anthropology and nursing. Today the team approach to the patient in pain may include a comparable variety of professionals—psychiatrists, internists, surgeons, neurologists, neurosurgeons, anesthesiologists, physical therapists, social workers and nurses. In this book we will attempt to identify and describe the nurse's role in the care of the patient with pain.

The word "pain" brings to mind an endless variety of feelings, sensations and situations. Silently recall your last painful experience and then ask a friend to tell you about his. There may be very little similarity between the two stories, except that both are about something unpleasant. For example, you may have remembered the sore throat you had last week, but your friend may have told you about how painfully sad it was to lose his pet dog. Hence, innumerable experiences can be described as painful.

In this first chapter we will define our use of the word "pain" in this book and explain how pain is relevant to nursing practice.

What human experiences are described as painful?

Most people use the word "pain" to refer to experiences that they find unpleasant and would like to avoid. To encompass these numerous meanings, pain can be conceptualized as occurring at both the bodily and mental levels. On both levels pain results from a breach in a protective barrier (Ramzy and Wallerstein). With bodily pain there is

1

an uncomfortable sensation that can be localized in some part of the body. For example, if the foot is cut by stepping on a piece of glass, an unpleasant sensation occurs that is localized in the sole of the foot. The continuity of the skin, one of the protective barriers of the body, is breached or invaded. With mental or nonbodily pain there is an uncomfortable feeling that is difficult to localize in any specific part or parts of the body. For example, the loss of a loved one can cause the unpleasant, generalized feelings associated with grief and mourning. In mental pain the protective barrier that is breached is psychic in nature, a loss or injury to the person's emotional wholeness. On both the bodily and mental levels pain serves to warn of danger. Bodily pain warns of the danger of physical harm; mental pain warns of the loss or threat of loss of something important to the person. Therefore, to summarize, those human experiences that are described as painful seem to have in common at least three factors: (1) a breach in a protective barrier or in the wholeness of the person, (2) a signal that warns of danger, and (3) an unpleasantness.

According to this conceptualization, mental pain includes not only the painful affects, or emotional experiences, of grief and mourning, fear, anxiety and guilt, but also painful ideas such as dreamed pain and the vivid remembrance of a physical pain. Bodily pain, as previously stated, includes all those unpleasant sensations that can be fairly well localized in some part of the body.

Considerable confusion has arisen as a result of attempts to classify bodily pain according to whether or not the pain sensation is initiated by a discernible physical stimulus. Bodily pain is commonly thought of as having some physical origin such as mechanical, chemical, electrical or thermal stimulation of the receptors in some part of the body. With some types of bodily pain these stimuli are not present initially or at all. This has led to the inaccurate conclusion that some pains are not "real." Many terms have been used erroneously in an effort to label pain that does not originate with a physical stimulus. The following discussion defines and differentiates between certain of these terms.

Bodily pain that does not originate with an identifiable physical stimulus traditionally has been called psychosomatic. Few terms are more confusing and more frequently misused than "psychosomatic." General usage of this word is meant to suggest either that the patient's illness and symptoms are totally imaginary, or that the patient's emotional problems are the cause of his physical illness. Usually the implication is that the patient should see a psychiatrist and that further physical ministrations are of little value. However, "psychosomatic" more accurately refers to an approach to the care of patients that encompasses the needs of the total human being, both psychological and physiological aspects.

No pain is truly imaginary. Some types of pain (and certain other symptoms) appear to originate solely from the mental or psychological state of the individual. However, the patient actually feels a sensation of pain; he is not merely thinking or imagining he has pain. Pain of psychological origin is usually called psychogenic or psychoneurotic. These terms include, among other conditions, hysteria (conversion reaction) and hypochondriasis. Phantom pain has also been included among these conditions. The localized sensation of pain that can occur with hysteria, hypochondriasis and phantom pain does not necessarily originate with a physical stimulus. Simply stated, the stimuli for these pains are thought to occur in the past experience of the person, seeming to involve long-standing inabilities to resolve emotional needs or conflicts. These stimuli breach the psychic boundaries rather than the bodily boundaries. But they do not cause painful emotions. Instead, they cause the localized sensation of pain at the bodily level.

In hysterical pain repression of conflicts is a major factor. An event causes the person to feel impelled to do something he has always wanted to do but felt he should not. He utilizes pain to repress the desires for which he feels guilty. For example, an adult male had harbored strong but conflicting love and aggression toward his father since early childhood. He suddenly developed severe pain in his arm during an argument with his father, because he wished to strike his father. The pain allowed him to repress this conflict; it prevented him from yielding to the desire to hit his father and also punished him for the temptation to do so. Such a mechanism is entirely unconscious and the patient is aware only of the resulting pain.

Hypochondriacal pain is thought to be based on past experiences that resulted in difficulty in establishing meaningful relationships with people. Actual physiological alterations at the site of the pain sensation may occur in the patient as a result of chronic emotional tension. However, the original stimulus for pain resides in the person's past experiences. Repeated failure to form close relationships with others results in withdrawal of emotional investment in people and reinvestment of this emotion in the person's own body. He becomes morbidly preoccupied with the state of his body and uninterested in his surroundings. The onset of hypochondriasis may be associated with a situation that threatens to weaken still further any relationships with others. Perhaps the patient is conditioned to experience pain when he is unable to relate meaningfully to others, or it may be that his tremendous emotional investment in his own body causes him to interpret sensations as painful when ordinarily such sensations would go almost unnoticed. For whatever the reason, the hypochondriac attempts on an unconcious level to adjust to his failure at relationships. Hypochondriacal pain, as described here, is rare. But, the term "hypochondriac" is used loosely and frequently refers to patients whom the staff find annoying because of their unending physical complaints.

Phantom pain, another relatively rare condition, involves the perception of pain in a part of the body that has been removed. The occurrence of phantom pain is most often associated with an amputated limb. Phantom pain has also been known to occur following removal of internal organs; for example, gastric ulcer pain may persist following gastrectomy. The mechanism for phantom pain has been described variously as an attempt to deny the loss of a body part (if it hurts it must still be there), as an underlying depression in which the person's anger over dependency needs that he finds unacceptable is turned inward on himself and takes the form of pain, as abnormal or painful stimuli from neuromas or scars (Sternbach, 1968), and more recently as decreased inhibition of impulses in the central nervous system (Melzack, 1970; b). Since patients with phantom pain often experience pain relief from measures designed to relieve depression, most authorities seem to believe that underlying depression is a major stimulus for the presence of this pain (Sternbach, 1968). If this is true, the mechanism underlying phantom pain is on an unconscious level as it is for hypochondriasis and hysteria.

In the preceding discussion of psychogenic or psychoneurotic pain, examples were given of conditions that possibly do not involve either a physical stimulus for the origin of the pain or any sustained physiological changes. Another category of potentially painful conditions are also either initiated by or potentiated by emotional conflicts, but in these conditions there are sustained structural changes in the tissues. Again we encounter the term "psychosomatic" being applied to such conditions, but they are more accurately termed organ neuroses or psychophysiological autonomic and visceral responses (Hofling and Leininger). In these organic diseases psychological factors are felt to play a major role in pathogenesis. Examples of these diseases are essential hypertension, peptic ulcer, migraine headaches, ulcerative colitis, and various skin disorders. The list continues to grow as we continue to increase our understanding of the interplay of psychological and physiological factors. Indeed the definition of organ neuroses applies to virtually every disease when the patient is viewed as a total person.

Painful sensations, then, may be initiated or sustained by factors other than physical stimuli. Other mechanisms underlying pain may involve solely psychological factors, or an interaction of psychological and physiological elements. These mechanisms are strictly unconscious; they are below the level of awareness and not within the immediate control of the individual. Hence, none of the bodily pains mentioned thus far have anything to do with the malingerer—that is one who deliberately deceives. The malingerer is consciously motivated. He does not by definition actually feel any physical sensation of pain. He knows that he does not have pain, he experiences no discomfort and he does not believe that he has pain, but he consciously chooses to tell others that he is in pain. He often fears that his lie will be detected.

Which types of pain will be discussed in this book?

The types of pain discussed in this book encompass all varieties of bodily pain whether or not the localized sensation is initiated by a discernible physical stimulus. Henceforth the word "pain" refers to all localized sensations of bodily pain. The discussion will not exclude what we have labeled mental pain, but mental pains such as anxiety and guilt will be considered only to the extent that they influence the patient's total pain experience.

Pain will be discussed in terms of the nursing care of the patient with pain. A very important assumption in this book is that the care of a patient with pain is best accomplished by attending to all physiological, sociocultural and psychological factors that affect his pain. Many of these factors will be discussed in relation to assessment, intervention and evaluation of the patient with pain. The discussion will include all age groups and will not be limited to any particular clinical setting. Not all that is said will apply equally well to all patients or all types of pain. This would be impossible since each patient with pain should be assisted in an individualized manner. But, hopefully, a careful consideration of the many methods for assessment, intervention and evaluation will yield an effective approach for any patient who has any type of pain.

Why is the study of pain relevant to the nurse?

The fear of pain is said to rank second only to the fear of death (Zborowski, 1969). And of course pain is often associated with death. Without question, pain is the most frequent and compelling reason why a person seeks medical assistance (Zborowski, 1969). Some patients come to the physician because of complaints other then pain, but they often anticipate that pain will occur in the course of diagnosis and treatment. Therefore, regardless of the clinical setting in which the nurse practices, she will have multiple and perhaps daily encounters with persons anticipating and experiencing pain, and pain will probably be of utmost concern to them.

Although pain brings the patient to the physician, usually the nurse is the person most consistently available to the patient during the long hours and days he experiences pain. At times the nurse may be the *only* person available to him. The critical importance of the nurse in treating pain has been noted by several physicians who have researched pain. With regard to postoperative pain, for example, it has been noted that the quality of nursing care exerts a definite influence on the frequency and severity of pain (Dodson and Bennett). Further, it has been suggested that physicians hold many misconceptions about the severity of postoperative pain because it is the nurse, not the physician, who treats postoperative pain (Keats). This is not to say that the nurse is the only person who does or should treat pain. Rather the nurse, who has more contact with the patient than any other member of the health team, is in a position to make invaluable contributions to any planned program of pain relief.

What are some differences between the nurse's and the physician's approaches to the patient with pain?

This section will identify two quite different approaches to the care of the patient with pain: the primarily physicalistic and the psychological. These approaches may be compared in terms of three aspects of the pain experience: the feeling of pain, the relationship of pain to the body and the method of verification of the pain (Szasz).

The physicalistic approach to the patient with pain is used, at least initially, by the physician because he is expected to make a physical diagnosis of the cause of the pain. He views pain as a sensation that has a somewhat predictable relationship to a noxious stimulus or to abnormal neurophysiological activity. The body is then viewed as a physiochemical mechanism in which a noxious stimulus is processed or in which abnormal physiological activity takes place. Implicit in all the diagnostic tests is the notion that the pain can be verified objectively. In other words, the physician checks on the complaint of pain by attempting to ascertain a cause for it. In much the same way as a physician determines whether or not a patient is sick, he also determines whether or not a patient *should* have pain. The effect of this on the patient can be exemplified by the two possible outcomes of the diagnostic measures, that is, positive or negative results. If the cause of the pain is found, the physician then gives the patient the findings of his diagnosis and explains why he experiences pain. In essence the physician has told the patient that the pain has been verified. But if no cause for the pain is found after several attempts at diagnosis, the patient may begin to think that the physician does not believe he has pain. Indeed, this may be the physician's opinion. Regardless of the physician's belief, he is put in the position of telling the patient after each series of diagnostic tests that he has not found anything wrong with him. This means, of course, that the physician does not yet understand why the patient has pain. However, the fact that the physician cannot verify the pain may raise several doubts and fears in the patient's mind. Patients who have had multiple diagnostic procedures with negative findings often remark that they are afraid the physician thinks there is actually nothing wrong with them and that the pain is imaginary. Many such patients say something to the effect of, "I know I'm not crazy. I don't see how it could be all in my mind. I really feel the pain." The patient may fear that the physician will abandon him if no cause can be found for the pain. While it may be essential for the physician to use the physicalistic approach, the results are unfortunate if it is utilized exclusively.

The nurse often contributes information about the patient that is important to the physician's physicalistic approach, but she is not responsible for making the physical diagnosis. Her primary and unique responsibility seems to lie more in the realm of assisting the patient to cope with pain regardless of the cause of the pain or whether the cause is known. The nurse may then use a predominantly psychological approach toward the patient. Using this approach, the patient's pain is viewed not as a sensation but as an affect, eliminating the idea that there will be a predictable relationship between noxious stimuli and the feeling of pain. The patient's experience of pain is seen as involving far more than a localized sensation; it encompasses what this sensation means to him. In an attempt to understand the meaning of his pain the patient's personal and social characteristics become important areas of assessment. The body in which this sensation of pain occurs cannot be viewed as a machine, but rather as the patient's personal, private possession, invested with that patient's particular emotions. An appreciation of the patient's conscious and unconscious perceptions of his body further enhances an understanding of pain as an emotional experience. With the conceptualization of pain as an affect, verification of the pain by others is meaningless. Pain can be verified only by the person experiencing it.

The use of this psychological approach by the nurse does not eliminate consideration of physical and physiological aspects of pain. However, it is not restricted to these aspects. It focuses on pain in the context of the total person and assumes that the experience of pain exists if the patient says that it does. The diagnostic measures and treatments done for the patient are not for the sole purpose of determining the cause of the pain, but for the purpose of finding some way to assist the patient in pain. For example, one practical application of this attitude is that the negative findings of a diagnostic test are reported to the patient in terms of being unable as yet to find another way to help him.

The nurse's psychological approach enables her to gain a greater understanding of the patient's pain experience so that she can intervene effectively on that level. Her intervention includes the management of both psychological and physiological factors. Communication of her observations and conclusions to other members of the health team assists them in understanding another aspect of the patient's care. Just as the nurse uses the physician's physical findings in determining intervention possibilities, the physician may use the nurse's assessment in his interactions with the patient and in making a physical diagnosis.

What definition of pain is most relevant to nursing practice?

No concise definition of pain will be adequate. However, a workable definition of pain is a useful way of getting oriented to the subject. Consequently, there are almost as many definitions of pain as there are writers on the topic. This author will offer still another one.

This book focuses on what nurses may contribute to the management of the patient with pain. Nurses are only one of several groups who attempt to assist the patient with pain. Therefore, an important criterion for our definition of pain is that it capitalize on what nurses can offer. Another essential criterion is that it should be maximally beneficial to the patient. To develop such a definition of pain we must first discard the notion that pain is simply and literally a localized sensation of hurt. *Pain is an abstract concept that refers to sensation, stimulus and response* (Sternbach, 1968). All of these aspects of pain must be attended to by all persons who contribute to the management of pain. The fundamental point of reference for the nurse's approach is the patient's subjective experience of pain, comprised of the patient's own perceptions of the situation (McBride, 1969). This is consistent with the psychological approach described previously and is broader than the strictly physicalistic approach. If the nurse's basic orientation to pain is the patient's subjective experience, all of her observations of the patient, on both the physiological and psychological levels, are relevant to her understanding of what the patient is experiencing. All the nursing interventions that result from this assessment are evaluated in terms of their effect on what the patient experiences from his own point of view.

Based on this type of approach to pain, a workable definition of pain for nurses can be very simply stated: *Pain is whatever the experiencing person says it is and exists whenever he says it does.* This definition is also beneficial to the patient because it is actually his definition. This utilizes the psychological approach and assumes that the patient is the only person who knows what he feels and when he feels it. Even if no physiological or psychological cause for pain is identified, the patient's report of pain is never doubted—the patient is always believed. This orientation has already been succinctly stated in the nursing literature as "real knowledge of what pain *is* belongs only to the one who experiences it" (Kaufmann and Brown, p. 48).

Our definition of pain stipulates that the patient "says" something to us about the pain. This term does not mean that the patient must verbalize. Many patients will not or cannot communicate verbally. What the patient says to us includes all voluntary and involuntary behaviors and all verbal and nonverbal behaviors. The next chapter discusses the numerous behaviors that may indicate the existence and characteristics of pain the patient experiences. A gasp and the rapid movement of the hand to the abdomen tell us that the patient's pain is probably sudden, located in the abdominal region, and of moderate to high intensity. The patient may indicate further that it is frightening or depressing, shown by his concern over the prognosis of his disease or his inability to go back to work and support his family. All of this and much more is part of what the patient says to us about his subjective experience of pain.

How will the nursing study of pain be approached?

Nursing is essentially an applied science. Therefore, when the nurse studies pain, she needs an approach that facilitates the application of knowledge to patient care. To accomplish this, a problem-solving approach to patient care is adopted in this book. Knowledge, theories and principles related to pain are systematically ordered in terms of this approach. Each of the first six chapters is an element of the problem-solving approach.

The actual use of the problem-solving approach in the care of patients is never as clear and precise as the chapter headings suggest. In the first place, problem-solving is a circular process in which evaluation is not the end but rather the beginning of another assessment of the problem. Secondly, the steps of problem-solving are rarely self-contained. The act of assessment may also be a form of intervention. For example, when the nurse talks to the patient about his pain experience for the purpose of obtaining information, she is also intervening. She is showing concern, reducing isolation of the patient by her presence, and reducing anxiety by helping him focus his attention.

Despite much overlap of the elements of problem-solving, they nevertheless exist and are useful ways of ordering information systematically. This is an aid to the learning and patient care processes. Studying a subject in depth is facilitated by breaking it down into its components according to some system. And caring for patients, especially those who are labeled complex and do not seem to respond to interventions suggested by experience and intuition, is often more effective if assessments of the patients are logically ordered for analysis and intervention.

Further Exploration

At the beginning of this chapter a broad conceptualization of pain was used to introduce the topic and to assist with definition of related terms. This model was a psychoanalytic one, but its clarity was the reason for choosing it. It may well be that a behavioral approach, or even a neurophysiological orientation, would be a better method of introducing nurses to a concept of pain. For example, classical conditioning is an excellent mechanism for understanding the interrelationships between unpleasant affects and bodily pain and for noting that either one may precipitate the other.

The suggested nursing approach to pain and the nursing definition of pain may also be questioned. They undoubtedly reflect a philosophy of nursing care, a philosophy which was not stated and which may not be shared by the reader. Many readers will want to determine at the outset whether or not the approach and definition are consistent with their own philosophies.

Another area of concern may have occurred to some readers, namely that the suggested nursing definition of pain entails treating the malingerer in the same manner as the patient who actually, consciously experiences pain. Some nurses more easily accept believing patients with pain originating with or sustained by the psychological state than they can accept equal treatment for the malingerer. However, there are relatively few malingerers. Detection of the malingerer may be complex and is not the nurse's responsibility, although her observations may assist in detection. It is true that this nursing definition of pain may aid the malingerer in accomplishing his goals, but the situation is somewhat analogous to the principles of our judicial system. A man is innocent until proven guilty beyond a reasonable doubt. This supposedly results in some guilty persons being freed, but fewer innocent ones are punished. Similarly, with our definition of pain, some lies will be believed, but the patient who experiences pain will never be doubted. Can you imagine the agony of someone in pain who can find no one to believe him? There are numerous such instances, some ending with tragic deaths due to undiagnosed disease.

Chapter | 2

Nursing Assessment of Patient Behaviors Related to the Pain Experience

Assessment is necessarily based upon a definition of what is being observed. The nursing definition of pain has been stated as being whatever the experiencing person says it is, existing whenever he says it does. It has been stipulated that what the patient says about pain involves far more than his verbalizations. Therefore assessment will be based on a variety of observable behaviors.

A comprehensive assessment is important because of several factors that complicate the acquisition of an understanding of the patient's pain experience. First, and obviously, it is impossible ever to know exactly what the patient is feeling no matter how much effort is exerted by both patient and nurse. But an assessment that is as complete as possible will help to narrow the gap between the patient's experience and the nurse's understanding.

Secondly, attention to observation of the patient's behaviors prevents a commonly occurring pitfall in the management of pain—the nurse's assumption that pain exists because an adequate physical stimulus is present. Numerous researchers have discovered not only that comparable lesions do no elicit comparable degrees of pain but, more importantly, that some people will report severe pain and others will report no pain at all even though the degrees of physical trauma are similar. Even upon direct questioning these patients deny pain and fail to show any other signs of it. We are not talking about people having a congenital or acquired insensitivity to pain, but about those who simply do not experience pain in a given situation. Even if the patient cannot communicate verbally, it is rarely necessary for the nurse to assume the presence of pain. Other behaviors may be observed that help to verify whether or not pain is experienced.

Thirdly, there are patients who experience pain but do not report it freely. Cultural expectations may dictate that the patient bear the pain in silence, or the patient may wish to keep his pain a secret because he fears the surgical or medical treatment for it. In such instances the nurse must be alert to the more involuntary behavioral indications of pain.

Fourthly, some patients are unable to communicate verbally. A language barrier may exist because the patient is a baby without symbolic language, a young child with limited language or an immigrant who speaks only a foreign language. With these patients the nurse must be able to recognize the presence of pain on the basis of patient behaviors other than verbalizations.

Since this guide to nursing assessment of the patient in pain relies entirely upon the patient's behaviors, it is important to have a clear definition of the term "behavior." In this book behavior will refer to all of the patient's voluntary or involuntary acts that can be observed directly or indirectly through the five senses (hearing, vision, touch, taste, smell) of another person.

Although observations of behaviors serve to assist the nurse in understanding the patient's *subjective* experience of pain, the behaviors themselves are *objective* evidence. Wherever possible, behaviors will be described objectively, so that more than one person will be able to make reliable observations of the patient and share them with others with the interjection of a minimum amount of personal bias. For example, the nurse may report that the patient seems worried about the meaning of his pain. She has reached a tentative conclusion based upon objective data that she should also report so that others can arrive at their own conclusions. The objective evidence may be: a blood pressure of 180/120; a wrinkling of the brow; and the patient's statement, "I don't know how I can live with this pain." With this type of data the nurse making the observations and those to whom she reports them are better able to confirm or oppose the original conclusion. Further evidence may suggest that this patient is not as concerned with the implications of his pain as he is with obtaining relief from it.

This discussion of patient behaviors will help the nurse to assess three aspects of the pain experience: (1) the fact that pain is present, (2) characteristics of the pain sensation such as intensity, location and duration and (3) the meaning of the pain experience to the patient. These observations are relevant to the three phases of the pain experience: (1) anticipation of pain, (2) the presence of pain and (3) the aftermath of pain. It is well known that the anticipation of pain may be a more difficult experience for the patient than the actual presence of pain. What happens during the period of anticipation profoundly affects responses to the presence of pain. The aftermath of pain has received less attention in the literature. But there is little doubt that it is an equally important phase of the pain experience and warrants as complete an assessment as the others.

Clearly, the objective assessment of the patient's behavioral responses to the pain experience serves a very practical purpose in the performance of nursing care activities. Once the assessment of the individual patient is made, the nurse knows that a particular group of behaviors may mean that this patient anticipates pain, experiences pain or has recently experienced pain. This alerts her to the need for nursing intervention. Knowledge of the characteristics of the pain and the meaning of the pain to the patient enables her to devise intervention specific to the patient's needs. Further, since she possesses knowledge of the patient's behavioral responses to the pain experience prior to her intervention, the assessment of behavioral responses after intervention enables her to evaluate the effectiveness of her nursing care.

To facilitate analysis of the nurse's assessment the patient's possible behavioral responses to the pain experience are divided into eight categories: (1) physiological manifestations, (2) verbal statements, (3) vocal behaviors, (4) facial expressions, (5) body movement, (6) physical contact, (7) general response to the environment and (8) patterns of handling pain. These categories of behavior are intimately related and each must be evaluated within the context of the total response of the patient. Consequently there will be some overlapping remarks in this discussion of the behaviors.

What are the physiological manifestations associated with pain?

Observation of the patient's physiological response to the pain experience is a useful aid in determining whether or not pain is present, duration of the pain, meaning of the pain in terms of the amount of anxiety accompanying the experience, and to a certain extent the intensity of the pain sensation. The nature of these involuntary physiological responses appears to be dependent upon at least two significant factors: the duration of the pain experience (that is, minutes versus days of pain) and the amount of anxiety associated with it. Apparently, when pain occurs in the absence of anxiety, the physiological responses are comparable to those occurring in the orienting reaction to any novel stimulus, involving only slight increases in heart rate, depth of respiration and palmar sweating (Shor). We will assume, however, that the pain experience of almost all patients will be accompanied by anxiety since people usually become patients because of some concern over their health. Physiological responses to pain will then be presented in terms of duration of the pain, adhering to the basic sequence and principles suggested by Sternbach's (1968) review of the literature.

Individual differences in response styles as well as numerous other factors such as variations in the pain sensation prohibit statements of the specific levels of physiological response and of the exact amount of time that will elapse before the response will change. It should also be noted that although the physiological responses generally will be stated in terms of the second phase of pain, that is, the presence of the pain sensation, the responses may also occur in the anticipation or aftermath phases.

Activation. The first pattern of physiological responses to pain is referred to as activation, and usually takes place within the first second or so of a rather sudden and intense pain sensation. If the pain continues, the responses may be sustained for a few minutes up to about an hour. Activation is also characteristic of anger and fear and it has often been called the "fight or flight reaction." [The original and classic description of these responses to a variety of conditions was done in 1929 by Cannon.] The physiological changes appear to be directly serviceable to the individual. They prepare him to defend himself or escape, a reaction necessary for the survival of the human race in a hostile environment.

During the period of activation the sympathetic nervous system is dominant. What the nurse most often observes in the patient is an increase in pulse and respiratory rates, increase in diastolic and systolic blood pressure, pallor, dilated pupils, increase in muscle tension or various body movements, cold perspiration and/or raised hairs in some areas of the body. The patient may report nausea or a "hollow stomach." These observations reflect a tremendous amount of physiological activity. Blood shifts from the viscera and superficial vessels, organs whose activities are deferrable, to the organs immediately essential to muscular exertion such as the striated muscles, lungs, heart and central nervous system. As a result, gastric secretions and contractions are inhibited. The bronchioles dilate to increase oxygenation of the blood and there is also an increase in the number of red blood cells. To combat fatigue, the circulating blood sugar increases through utilization of carbohydrate stored in the liver. The vigor of cardiac contraction increases, facilitating distribution of the enriched blood supply. The danger of bleeding is minimized by circulating adrenalin and a decreased coagulation time. These sympathetic nervous system activities are sustained by the secretion of adrenalin which mimics sympathetic activity. Recently some investigators (Masuda and Dudley) noted that the responses to pain include not only an increase in respiratory rate but also an increase in alveolar ventilation and oxygen consumption and a decrease in alveolar carbon dioxide concentration.

Rebound. The next set of responses depends upon the duration and intensity of the pain sensation that initiated activation. If the original sensation was brief but intense the phenomenon of rebound may occur. These responses are the opposite of activation; they are like parasympathetic responses and are usually of short duration. The nurse may observe rebound responses by noting in the aftermath of pain that the pulse rate is slower than it was before pain occurred or that the blood pressure is lower than it was prior to pain. The compensatory reflexes stimulated during activation outlast the sympathetic responses.

Adaptation. Adaptation occurs if the stimulus for activation is repetitive or of long duration. The extreme physiological activity of activation cannot continue indefinitely, but it may take some time, several hours, before the responses of adaptation can be observed. They are compensatory responses that are stimulated by the prolonged sympathetic responses. Adaptation is actually a decrease in the sympathetic responses and the nurse can observe that there is less of an increase in the pulse rate and the blood pressure. In other words, as time goes on there is a decrease in the magnitude of response to pain. The exact mechanism underlying adaptation is not completely understood but may be related to antagonistic innervation, sympathetic inhibition and/or central inhibition at the spinal level.

Stress Reaction. The general adaptation syndrome, or stress reaction, occurs when pain or another stressor persists for days or many hours (Selye, 1946, 1956). While activation responses rely largely on autonomic innervation, the general adaptation syndrome depends upon hormonal reactions. These are more difficult responses for the nurse to observe, but she may note in the final stage of the stress reaction that tests reveal a greater production of 17-ketosteroids than 17-hydroxycorticosteroids and an increase in circulating eosinophiles, and that the physician's case history and physical analysis suggests various degenerative changes and an increased susceptibility to infections. Such findings are a result of the organism's inability to sustain a corticoid production sufficient to maintain resistance.

What is the nature of the verbal statements?

The patient's verbal statements about his pain may be none or many. Before describing this range of verbal behaviors it is important to consider how the patient's cognitive ability influences what he says. Cognitive ability involves how a person thinks and is the extent to which the individual organizes what he knows. In other words, it is the extent to which he possesses symbols of reality and manipulates them internally. Language is a symbolic means of communication. Thus a person's cognitive ability, irrespective of age, is one determinant of the existence of language and the effectiveness of language as a means of communication. For instance, the very young child below the age of about two years is unable to utilize language to convey his thoughts and feelings. On the other hand, it is easy to be misled by the language of a four- or five-year-old child. At this age the child usually has a large vocabulary and may be able to construct organized sentences. This barrage of language encourages the listener to believe that he understands what the child is saying. But a careful listener will find that the child often contradicts himself, that he fails to see or understand important aspects of a given topic, and that the meanings he ascribes to words are not necessarily those shared by adults.

When the adult's cognitive level is altered he may exhibit the same lack of verbal ability seen in the infant or the language difficulties of the young child. The adult's cognitive ability may be limited by many conditions such as brain damage or a lowering of the level of consciousness with drugs. Thus it should be understood that *the language problems encountered with the child may also occur in the adult.*

The importance of communication. A vast amount of information can be obtained from a patient who can communicate effectively and who will or can be encouraged to do so. The reliability of what the patient, especially the adult, says about his pain is attested to by the numerous researchers who have used this method to quantify pain and measure pain relief (Loan and Dundee, 1967; a). Some researchers (Zimbardo *et al.*) have also found that what the patient says about his pain is commensurate with the physiological measures. Since a nurse who is adept at communication skills can easily obtain statements about pain from an articulate patient and since these verbalizations appear to be highly reliable, nursing assessment of the patient in pain can justifiably rely heavily upon what the patient says. The patient's verbalizations, however, are subject to evaluation in terms of the influencing factors discussed in the next chapter.

What the patient's verbalizations may reveal about his pain can be broken down into several elements to assist the nurse in extracting information from what the patient volunteers and to assist her in interviewing the patient. These elements may be thought of as: the presence of pain; severity of the pain; tolerance for pain; quality, location, duration and rhythmicity of the pain; factors affecting the pain; and the meaning of the pain.

Presence, severity and tolerance of pain. The mere presence of pain may not be volunteered by the patient. If the nurse asks the patient if he has pain in his leg, his reply, "Well, I have a little discomfort," communicates something quite different from the voluntary remark, "My leg is really hurting." Differentiating between the presence, severity and tolerance of pain assists the nurse in obtaining useful information from these responses.

The presence of pain is sometimes referred to as pain threshold or pain perception threshold, defined as the least intensity of stimulus necessary to produce pain. Hence, when the intensity of a stimulus reaches the pain perception threshold, pain is present. Some research studies have defined pain perception threshold as the point at which *instructed* subjects first report graded exposures to noxious stimulation as painful (Wolff and Wolf). This suggests that the presence of very mild pain may not be mentioned by the patient unless he is asked to report it. Therefore, severity of pain is an important aspect of the pain assessment.

An effective method of determining the severity of pain is to ask the patient to rate his pain in some way. The nurse may tell the patient that she will be asking him from time to time to rate his discomfort as none, slight, moderate or intense (Loan and Dundee, 1967; a) or as none, a little bit, some, quite a bit or a lot (Lasagna). Helping the patient to rate his pain is pertinent to intervention, and using the same rating scale consistently is especially useful in evaluation.

The patient's rating of the severity of the pain does not necessarily indicate whether or not he wants something done to relieve the pain. The nurse must assess his tolerance for pain. Pain tolerance can be defined as the maximum intensity or duration of pain the person is willing to endure (Sternbach, 1968). Some patients may feel that it is senseless to experience even the mildest form of pain if something can be done about it. Other patients will not want anything done about severe pain. In the hospital setting the fact that the patient calls for the nurse and tells her about his pain usually implies that he has reached his tolerance level regardless of how he rates the severity of the pain. At that point he wants something done about his pain; he does not want to tolerate it any longer.

The following interaction is an example of how pain presence, severity and tolerance can be assessed. Mrs. Carter was admitted for reevaluation of degenerative arthritis because of increasing back pain. While the nurse was assisting Mrs. Carter with brushing her teeth, the nurse assessed the presence of pain by asking, "How is your back this morning?" Mrs. Carter replied, "It does bother me." The nurse responded, attempting to assess severity, "Oh, I'm sorry about that. Could you tell me if it is a little bit, some, quite a bit or a lot? As I mentioned yesterday it helps me understand how you feel if you can rate your discomfort this way." The patient answered, "Yes, I remember. I would say this is some pain." To assess tolerance the nurse asked, "Would you like something to be done about the discomfort?" Mrs. Carter replied, "No, not now. Later it will be worse and I'd like to save my treatments until then." This indicates that the patient thought she would reach her tolerance level later in the day as the pain increased.

Naturally, it is not as easy to obtain such precise information from a child. The child is sometimes unable to find the right words. He may have experienced the pain of a cut knee and said, "It hurts." But when he is faced with the new and strange experience of wound pain, he may not be able to understand that this is another form of pain to which the word "hurt" also applies (McCaffery, 1969). One four-year-old boy on the evening of his appendectomy was lying quietly in bed, perspiring, wide-eyed and frowning. The nurse approached him and asked, "Do you hurt?" He shook his head to indicate "No," but the nurse stayed with him a while and repeated the question. He was silent for several seconds before he moved his hand toward his abdomen and looked up at her to say, "Hurt? Hurt. Yes." Sometimes the presence of pain in a younger child is indicated only by his calling for his mother or father.

Characteristics of Pain. The quality of pain may be included in the patient's attempt to describe the severity of his pain. Theoretically there are supposed to be three pain qualities: pricking, burning and aching (Hardy, Wolff and Goodell, 1952; a). But patients use many other words to refer to pain and to explain how it feels. The word "pain" is not as frequently used by patients as one would think, and Keele suggests that this word is reserved for uncomfortable sensations that evoke emotion. Following is a partial list of other words that patients may use to denote the quality of pain. The nurse may also use these terms to ask the patient about his pain, since some patients are remarkably unable to describe pain.

jabbing	shooting	pressure	spasm
gnawing	stinging	hurt	contraction
stabbing	pinching	knife-like	hot (burning)
cramping	stretching	sharp	discomfort
throbbing	constricting	bright	sore
pulling	cutting	dull	vise-like

Other characteristics of pain are its location, duration and rhythmicity. The location of pain includes the body part, the extent of the area and how deep or superficial it is. Many patients do not report the location of pain because they assume the nurse knows or they think this information is relevant only to the physician in making his diagnosis. But location of pain is pertinent to nursing intervention, as the following example illustrates. During the second day after his abdominal surgery one patient requested medication for his abdominal pain. The nurse asked him to show her exactly where the pain was and she discovered that adhesive tape had excoriated and pinched the skin in the area pointed out by the patient.

Unfortunately children are less able to localize their pain. Following extensive surgery a child often will refrain from moving even a finger, as if he thought the pain involved his whole body. A child who cuts his hand frequently refuses to move the entire arm. And because children do not have a complete concept of their body parts, a child may tell you that his mouth hurts when the pain is obviously located in his red and raw throat.

Duration of pain is also difficult for children to identify because of their undeveloped concept of time. Adults may be able to tell the nurse approximately how many minutes, hours or days they have had a particular pain. When someone is unable to state how long the pain has lasted, it is often possible for the nurse to help the patient associate the onset of pain with a particular event. One patient who did not have a watch told the nurse that he had been experiencing pain for about three hours. When she asked him when it had begun he said that it was after lunch. Since it was 1:30 p.m. and the nurse knew he had finished his lunch at 12:30, she was able to determine more accurately the duration of the pain.

To determine rhythmicity of the pain the nurse can ask the patient not only how long this pain has lasted but how often it occurs and whether or not the intensity varies. This is relevant to the timing of certain nursing interventions and may be useful data for the physician. Many types of pain such as arthritis, postoperative wound pain and headaches wax and wane under the influence of numerous factors.

Factors affecting the pain are often related to its rhythmicity and severity. Nursing intervention is determined in part on the basis of what seems to cause the pain and what the patient believes has helped relieve it. These factors affecting pain are so numerous it is possible to mention only a few of them. They may involve pressure, movement, position, eating and what is eaten, fatigue or coughing. The patient may believe that he obtains pain relief from morphine injections or some popular commercial preparation, from drinking milk or eating prunes, from lying perfectly still or running around the block. Many of these factors are discussed in the next chapter, but because they are frequently a part of the patient's verbalizations about pain they are also included here.

The meaning of pain is an extremely important aspect of the pain experience and this too is discussed in the following chapter. But, again, part of the patient's verbalizations about pain may include the significance of his pain to him. The nurse may note the extent to which pain causes the patient to be concerned about his prognosis, obtaining pain relief, going back to work, loneliness and many other possibilities.

Finally, in addition to noting what the patient says, the tone of voice and speed of speech should be observed. A high level of anxiety may be revealed by rapid and high pitched speech, or intense pain may be indicated by slow and monotonous speech. Anger is often implicit in loud staccato speech.

What are the vocalizations?

Vocalizations refer to all those emitted sounds that are not language, or at least cannot be understood as words by others. Patients who can verbalize may also use vocal behaviors to indicate the presence, severity, duration or meaning of pain. Vocalizations include groaning, grunting, whimpering, whining, crying, sobbing, screaming, gasping and many others. Some of these sounds are practically involuntary if the pain is sudden, sharp and unexpected. Such pain often elicits a gasp, a grunt or even a scream.

Some adults, because of cultural expectations, will not have as many vocalizations as other adults or children. For children, however, who do not have great facility with language, vocalizations may be an important means of communication. This may be the child's only way to inform others that he is in pain and needs their assistance (McCaffery, 1969).

Objective assessment of vocalizations entails description of pitch and loudness and notations of frequency and duration. A particular patient may cry in many ways. He may cry softly at low pitch for about 25 seconds five to six times a day and he may also cry loudly at low pitch for about 5 seconds once a day.

What are the facial expressions?

The patient's facial expression may be the first or the only sign of pain, or facial expressions may accompany a variety of other behaviors. When a patient does not verbalize or vocalize, facial expression may be an excellent indication of his pain experience. Some patients may have a rather normal and sober expression such as opened eyes and no wrinkling of the skin in any part of the face. Others may have clenched teeth, tightly shut lips, widely opened or tightly shut eyes, wrinkled forehead, biting of the lower lip, spreading of the lips and tightening of the muscles in the jaw or any number of other facial contortions.

As with vocalizations, facial expressions may indicate presence, severity, duration and meaning of pain. They may be almost involuntary at times, and they should be objectively described, taking into account frequency and duration.

What is the amount and type of body movement?

The amount and type of body movement may give clues to the

presence, severity, duration, location and meaning of pain. There are four predominant types of body movement accompanying the pain experience: immobile, purposeless or inaccurate, protective, and rhythmic or rubbing. Frequency and duration of these movements should be noted.

Immobilization means that the patient sustains one particular position for either a part of the body or the total body. Patients often do this to minimize their pain. It has already been mentioned that young children tend to immobilize the total body down to the little finger following massive physical trauma. Small injuries to a portion of a limb often result in their failing to move the whole limb. Adults are particularly reluctant to move the first few hours after abdominal or thoracic surgery. This reluctance to move may also occur after some accidental injuries that potentially involve many parts of the body or that may have resulted in life-threatening trauma. Patients may sustain whatever position they happen to be in. Or, they may purposely choose a position of maximum comfort such as a horizontal position for a spinal headache or a semi-Fowler's position after cholecystectomy. Apparently even infants draw up their legs in response to abdominal cramping although they do not tend to remain in this position. Following thoracic surgery the patient may limit all movement to prevent the need to breathe deeply or rapidly because of the pain of moving the chest wall. Any patient who immobilizes only a small part of his body gives the nurse a fairly good indication of the location of his pain. In fact, generalized lack of movement may also indicate location as well as quality of pain. The influence of pricking cutaneous and aching visceral pain upon body movement is discussed in the next chapter, the latter being associated with lack of movement. Thus, a child with a distended bladder may be relatively inactive compared to a child whose hand has been burned.

During any type of voluntary immobilization the muscles may be relaxed or tense, and this is important to note. There is generally some amount of muscle tension, such as the easily observed clenched fist, but through experience some patients know that relaxation minimizes pain and they will attempt to do this. The patient trained in the Lamaze method is an excellent example of this since her muscles may remain completely relaxed throughout labor.

The purposeless or inaccurate body movements that may accompany pain may be due to the excess energy usually occurring at the onset of severe pain, trembling, fear, or the patient's inability to find any way to help himself. The patient may flail his arms, kick, or toss and turn in bed. Purposeful motions sometimes become inaccurate during pain such as reaching for a glass and knocking it over.

The goal of protective movements associated with pain is to prevent the occurrence of pain or its increase. These movements may take the form of consciously controlled flight reactions for which the initial physiological processes so aptly prepare the person. Or, protective movements may be reflex responses, which are involuntary movements executed without conscious effort. Reflex responses, of course, are a type of flight reaction. However, we will differentiate between flight reactions that are largely voluntary and those that are not. Voluntary flight reactions may range from literally running away from a threat of pain to careful shielding of the threatened part using the hands or objects. A child who is threatened with a venipuncture may get out of bed and try to leave the room or he may hug his arms to his body and lie down on them. An adult may splint his incision with a pillow before he turns from side to side.

The involuntary, reflexive reactions also occur in both adults and children. Adults, however, are more likely to attempt to control reflexive responses. The neurophysiological processes underlying the reflex response can be summarized in the following example. When the hand touches a hot object it is swiftly withdrawn. In terms of the reflex arc a series of events occur in a fraction of a second, Receptors in the skin are stimulated by the hot object. Nerve impulses flash over the dendrite, cell body and axon of the afferent neuron into the dorsal horn of spinal gray matter. The nerve impulse then crosses the synapse between the axon of the afferent neuron and the dendrite of a central neuron. The impulse continues along the dendrite, the cell body and the axon of this central neuron. The impulse then crosses another synapse to the dendrite of an efferent neuron in the ventral horn of spinal gray matter. Continuing along the dendrite, the cell body and the axon of this motor neuron, the nerve impulse reaches the motor end plate in a skeletal muscle. This activates the contractile protoplasm and enables the person to withdraw from the painful stimulus (Chaffee and Greisheimer). During a bone marrow biopsy an adult may involuntarily jump away slightly when there is sudden pricking or extreme pressure. He may apologize and consciously attempt to react in opposition to this reflexive movement the next time it occurs. A child who jumps away may be unwilling or unable to exert any control over the reflex response.

Patients with pain frequently utilize some type of rhythmic or rubbing body movements. A baby may rub his ear if he has otitis media. When he is teething he is in effect rubbing his swollen gums as he chews on an object. With a headache an adult or young child may rub his head. Rocking in a semi-fetal position is common with abdominal or uterine cramping. During labor the Lamaze patient, because of her training, may employ "effleurage," a rhythmic massage of the abdomen with both hands. Rubbing or rhythmic movements may be excellent clues as to the location of pain.

How is physical contact with others utilized?

The patient not only responds to his own body with touch, position or movement during the pain experience, but in the process of interacting with another person will indicate his interest in physical contact from a source outside himself. His use of physical contact with others reveals much about the meanings and emotions associated with his pain experience such as varying degrees of anger, dependency and fear. In general this physical contact can be observed as fight reactions, initiation of touch, or passive or active acceptance of touch. Again, the type, frequency and duration should be noted.

The patient's initial physiological responses to pain typically prepare him for the flight reactions (previously discussed) or fight reactions. One way of fighting pain or the threat of pain is quite literally to attack the person who seems responsible for inflicting the pain. This aggressive physical contact can be seen in the child who kicks, hits, pushes away or bites the physician or nurse who approaches him with something he believes will induce pain. This occurs with less frequency and vigor in the adult, but an adult, for example, may push away the physician's hand if he palpates a tender liver.

Touch may be initiated by both adults and children. Many children want to be held during some phase of a pain experience. They may cling to any part of another person's body. An adult lying in bed helpless and in pain may reach out for the nurse the moment he sees her.

When the patient does not initiate touch, the nurse may offer it in the form of holding the patient's hand or rubbing some area of his body. The patient may accept this passively or actively. The patient demonstrates passive acceptance, for example, when he allows the nurse to hold his hand but does not actually grip her hand in return. Active acceptance would involve gripping her hand, or if she is stroking his forehead he might turn his head so that she can reach him more easily.

What is the general response to the environment?

Pain tends to draw attention to itself so that the patient is often preoccupied with pain during all phases of his pain experience. His interaction with the environment, including both objects and people, may drop to a minimum. It is important to observe the nature, extent, frequency and duration of this. He may fail to notice the flowers sent by a friend or that his extremities now wear the leads to a cardiac monitor. His social responses may involve withdrawal from people or a change in his communication patterns. He may no longer initiate conversation, or he may fail to respond when spoken to or give only short responses. Aside from the feelings of the pain experience, he may focus only on his body and those things done to him which might affect his pain.

Mrs. Anderson, forty years old, demonstrates this decrease in attention to the surrounding environment. The patient was at home recovering from a radical mastectomy. Minor contractures had developed because of her reluctance to perform the prescribed arm exercises. She was sitting on her porch talking enthusiastically with her husband and sister when the public health nurse arrived to assist her with the arm exercises. When Mrs. Anderson saw the nurse she immediately stopped talking. Until the exercises were completed she initiated no conversation and responded to no one except the nurse. Her husband and sister were standing a few feet away from the nurse and Mrs. Anderson. However, when Mr. Anderson suggested to his wife that she begin with the arm-swinging exercise since it was the least painful to her, she did not begin this until the nurse repeated the suggestion. Beginning with the anticipation of pain, Mrs. Anderson stopped talking and began focusing on the pain. Her attention was narrowed to the point that she seemed not to hear her husband's suggestion regarding the exercise. She attended only to the nurse, who seemed most related to the pain experience.

Has the patient developed a pattern of handling his pain?

Cultural expectations and the patient's own personal experience frequently enable him to develop a pattern of handling pain. Such a pattern involves a complex of behaviors that the patient tends to exhibit repeatedly. Therefore, this pattern may encompass any one or combination of behaviors previously discussed. Sometimes these patterns of behavior are referred to as adaptive mechanisms, coping behaviors or defense patterns. Regardless of how effective they are for the patient, they usually represent his best effort to cope with pain. They are especially pertinent for the nurse to observe.

Any of the usual defense mechanisms may be reflected in the behavior, such as denial of pain, intellectualization of pain, or projection of the pain onto someone else. For example, a patient with a long history of a bleeding and painful peptic ulcer may intellectualize his pain by reading books and articles on the subject. He may consistently use medical terminology to describe each occurrence of pain and the usual treatment for it. Children frequently use a combination of denial and projection in the aftermath phase of the pain experience. The following conversation took place in the hospital room between the nurse and Randy, five years old, and Paul, eight years old. It was the tenth day after Randy's open heart surgery and Paul's third day of hospitalization for treatment of an infected injury to the leg. The nurse began the conversation with Randy by asking him several times what had happened to him in the hospital. Randy persisted with replies such as "nothing" or shaking his head. When the nurse pointed to his incision and repeated her question Randy replied, "Oh, yes, I got that." When the nurse asked him if he had received injections he admitted this but upon direct questioning denied that they hurt. He then turned to Paul in the next bed and said, "But he cried when he got a shot." Both claimed that "shots" did not hurt, but an argument ensued between the two boys. Each claimed that he did not cry with the injection but that the other had cried. Both children denied that they experienced pain and projected their pain experience onto the other. Because Randy used denial with both the pain of surgery and injections, this may have been a pattern for him.

Other patterns of handling pain may be expressions of anger, powerlessness, fear or guilt. The powerless patient may respond with irritability, demands, and efforts to control others. He may be quite aware of his behavior and may be concerned about it, believing that his mental well-being is jeopardized by pain (McBride, 1969). No doubt many nurses have encountered at least one patient with a marked need to control others. Often he seems to have learned to anticipate the nurse's actions for the sole purpose of being able to order her to do whatever she had intended to do.

Body movements and vocalizations may be the outstanding pattern of handling pain in other patients. Some patients habitually rock and moan with pain. Others curl up in the fetal position and weep.

Further Exploration

Physiological responses. One physiological response to pain not previously discussed because the necessary equipment is not often used with patients in pain is the galvanic skin response (GSR). GSR is a drop in the skin's electrical resistance, measured in ohms. Several researchers have reported decreases in skin resistance in response to pain (e.g., Engel, Barber and Hahn, Shor). One nursing study found that GSR and heart rate changed in magnitude in response to labor contractions in both minimal and intense pain (Riehl). Alexander found that skin resistance changes distinguished between conditioned and unconditioned, and psychogenic and physical pain responses. He pointed out the importance of this from the standpoint of the patient's medical treatment since the physician must detect and treat the pathophysiology and secure appropriate psychiatric assistance with the psychogenic pain.

Although Riehl found the heart rate changes increased in magnitude in relation to the amount of pain, it appeared from her data that increased heart rate is more reliable as an indicator of the presence of pain. Sternbach (1966) also reports that heart rate as well as blood pressure increases are not reliable measures of the amount of pain experienced. Masuda and Dudley did not even find significant changes in the mean heart rate in response to noxious stimuli to the head.

Variability of response factors. Variable findings are reported for the physiological responses to pain and this is due to many factors of which the nurse, especially the researcher, may wish to be aware. Two of these factors are response-stereotypy among individuals and the law of initial values (Sternbach, 1966, 1968). Individuals have different physiological response styles. One person may always respond with maximum heart rate changes while another responds with maximum blood pressure changes. With regard to the law of initial values, the higher the prestimulus level of functioning, the smaller the magnitude of response to pain. In fact the direction of response, such as the tendency for the heart rate to increase rather than decrease, may change if the prestimulus level of functioning is higher than the response to pain. In this case the response to pain may be a decrease in physiological functioning such as a decrease in heart rate.

Pain measurement. This chapter discusses the use of observable behavioral responses for detecting and understanding the patient's pain experience. The nurse researcher may be interested in other methods of measuring pain. The most famous of these seems to be the Hardy-Wolff-Goodell dolorimeter. The dolorimeter is designed to deliver measured thermal radiation per unit area of skin. The intensity of this pricking pain is measured by a 10 point dol scale, 1 being just above the pain perception threshold. Each dol is 2 just noticeable differences (jnd's) in the level of pain intensity. Using the same principles this group designed the algesimeter to measure the aching pain of pressure on subcutaneous tissue. The findings of this group suggest that the intensities of aching and pricking pain can be compared, and change in the quality of pain does not alter the pain-intensity relationship. Further, the stimulus for pain can be increased in destructive power but will not evoke pain of any greater intensity than that perceived at the top of the dol scale (Hardy).

Another method of pain measurement compares a measured stimulus with pain of pathological origin. The patient attempts to equate these two sensations, giving a quantitative expression of pain severity. One technique is thymometry in which a noise signal of gradually increasing and measured intensity is compared with clinical pain. The instrument goes from 0 to 92 decibels. The originator of this method says that an ordinary clinical audiometer can also be utilized (Peck). Another apparatus has been designed in which pathologic pain is measured by the amount of air pressure needed to produce equal experimental pain (Kast).

Pain perception threshold. Controversy exists over this threshold concerning whether or not it varies from one person to another or within the same person. This deserves comment if for no other reason than that volumes of literature have been devoted to the subject. Under optimal conditions of measurement and training Hardy, Wolff and Goodell (1943, 1952; a, b) have demonstrated the uniformity of pain perception threshold between individuals and on all skin surfaces. Other studies, however, have failed to confirm this (e.g., Clark and Bindra, Schamp and Schamp). Beecher, (1956; a), an avid critic of the Hardy, Wolff and Goodell findings, believes that one reason why others fail to report uniformity of this threshold is that central processing of the sensation occurs before awareness of the sensation. For example, the person's memories of painful events are activated before a sensation reaches the level of awareness. Thus, memories influence the perception of the sensation before the person is conscious of experiencing pain. At any rate it is doubtful that the uniformity of the pain perception threshold, if it does exist, has any relationship with the pain experience of patients. On the other hand, the variability of pain reaction threshold, involving the individual's total responses to pain, is well established. It does not enjoy the controversy surrounding pain perception threshold.

Chapter | 3

Nursing Assessment of Factors Influencing the Patient's Behavior and the Pain Sensation

When a patient indicates that he is experiencing pain by exhibiting any one or combination of the behaviors discussed in the last chapter, the nurse makes a comprehensive and objective assessment of all his behaviors related to the pain experience. The next step in the nurse's problem-solving journey is to determine why the patient behaves in this way and to understand why he experiences a sensation of pain. She makes her own assessment and also uses data from the physician's findings. Those elements that affect the patient's sensation of pain or his response to pain are called influencing factors. In this chapter they are categorized as physiological and physical, cultural, and psychological.

To appreciate how any one influencing factor may affect both the sensation of pain and the behavioral response to it, a diagram of the interplay of stimulation, sensation and reaction, or behavior, is presented in Table 1 on the following page. This complex but basically circular interplay of biological, psychological and social responses during the pain experience shows how a factor that influences any part of the process will eventually affect the other components as well.

What are the physiological and physical factors influencing the patient's behavior and the pain sensation?

The physiological and physical factors presented here include: the neurophysiological processes underlying the sensation of pain; duration and intensity of pain; alterations in the level of consciousness; cutaneous versus visceral sites of pain; environmental conditions; sensory restriction; and physical strain and fatigue. The nature of the

Table 1. Interplay of responses during the pain experience.*

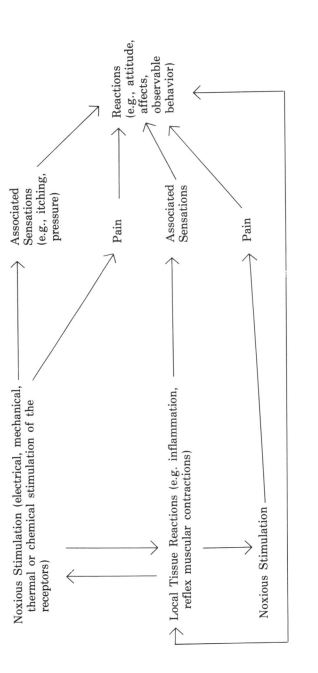

*Adapted from Hardy, 1956, p. 46.

stimulus capable of producing pain is referred to in the discussion of several of these factors. But it will become clear from the discussions throughout this chapter that there is not a direct and invariant relationship between any stimulus and the perception of pain. In other words, a given stimulus may or may not be perceived as painful. Even if it is perceived as painful, the same stimulus may cause pains of varying intensities. Therefore, the focus will not be on a systematic analysis of categories of noxious or pain-producing stimuli. The nurse is urged to identify the pain-producing stimulus in the individual patient by applying her knowledge of cultural and psychological influences as well as physiological and physical factors. In this section of physiological and physical factors two sources of noxious stimuli, environmental conditions and physical strain, are considered, however, because they are relevant to nursing intervention in that they may both cause pain and increase the intensity of an already existing pain sensation.

Neurophysiological processes underlying the sensation of pain. One way to understand why a person experiences pain is to identify the neurophysiological processes. Certain processes underlie the transformation of a stimulus into a sensation of pain with accompanying behavioral responses. Regardless of the originating stimulus for pain, whether it is mostly physical or psychological, all pain is physiological in the sense that physiological processes are necessary for the production of the pain sensation. This section, however, will deal mostly with those pain sensations that originate with or are sustained by more or less identifiable physical stimuli.

The fact that specific neuroanatomical structures are involved in the transformation of a noxious stimulus into felt pain does not necessarily explain *how* the sensation of pain is produced, any more than enumerating the muscles used in running explains how a man runs the mile in four minutes. Further, pain is not always felt when a noxious stimulus is transmitted over these neural pathways, and pain may be felt even when certain parts of the neuroanatomy are not functioning. The neuroanatomy of pain is somewhat analogous to a road map that shows the route from stimulus-City A to felt-pain-City B. Impulses may start at stimulus-City A and arrive at felt-pain-City B using a route altogether different from the one on the map. It is also possible that blocking one of the pathways will prevent the impulses from arriving at felt-pain-City B, or they may arrive by traveling alternate routes. Nevertheless, it is possible to outline the probable sequence of neural pathways traveled by most noxious stimuli.

When a noxious stimulus is applied to the skin of the leg, for example, receptors are stimulated. The impulse is carried by nerve fibers in the peripheral sensory nerves. These nerves are composed of a bundle of fibers that carry other impulses such as temperature changes and pressure. The sensory nerve fibers enter the dorsal root ganglia, each ganglion being a clump of cell bodies. From here the impulse travels to the dorsal horn of the spinal cord, crosses over to the opposite side of the spinal cord by way of the anterior commissure, and then upward by way of the lateral spinothalamic tracts to the thalamus. Here pain is perceived. The impulses are then projected to the sensory cortex where the perception of pain is interpreted and the behavioral responses such as flight or complaint are initiated.

There are some exceptions to this pathway for pain impulses, a few of which are mentioned here. Some of the fibers do not cross over and enter the lateral spinothalamic tract. Also, not all fibers project directly to the thalamus. Some fibers project to the reticular formation in the brain stem, and of these some project to the thalamic nuclei and some send impulses back down to cord cells. This projection of impulses back to the cord before reaching the thalamus where pain is perceived means that thresholds for response to incoming stimuli can be altered before perception of pain occurs. Further, it is possible for pain responses to occur in the absence of adequate activity in the structures between and including the receptors and thalamus (Sternbach, 1968).

Based on the notion that certain neuroanatomical structures are involved if not essential in the production of pain, many surgical procedures have been designed to alleviate pain. This is done by destroying a structure and interrupting the pain pathways. This may be achieved by surgical incision that completely and permanently divides the pathway or by stereotaxic methods using electrical, chemical, ultrasonic or radioactive measures for the destruction of nuclei and pathways. On a temporary basis some of the procedures can be done using local anesthetics. For control of chronic pain or the pain during surgery, local anesthetics such as procaine may be injected into the intrathecal space (spinal block), the epidural space (epidural nerve block), peripheral somatic nerves (regional block), the autonomic nerves such as the cervical sympathetic chain or the lumbar paravertebral sympathetic chain, or other areas. When these procedures are deliberately and accurately performed to produce temporary or permanent pain relief, they unfortunately sometimes fail. For example, the patient may continue to experience pain after a chordotomy, or the pain may return after only a brief period of time.

The discussion thus far has outlined the sequence of neuroanatomical structures that frequently seem to be involved when pain is felt. Two important questions now arise. First, why are some impulses felt as pain rather then some other sensation such as itching or pressure? The significance of this question is difficult to grasp initially because we are accustomed to assuming that a laceration, for example, will naturally result in pain. To explain that the impulses travel over certain neural pathways does not really explain why or how the impulses produce the sensation of pain. Secondly, why does the destruction of certain neuroanatomical structures sometimes succeed and sometimes fail to alleviate pain?

Current theories regarding the pain mechanism.   Currently there are three popular theories about the pain mechanism that provide some possible answers to these questions. These are the specificity theory, the pattern theory and the gate control theory, the latter being the most recently formulated. None of these adequately explains all sensations of pain, and all continue to be the subject of much debate. The three theories are presented here with the hope that one or the other of them will offer an adequate explanation for most pain sensations.

The specificity theory is the most orthodox view of pain. This model suggests that there is a pain modality that can be stimulated only by painful stimuli and, therefore, these impulses are always felt as pain and only as pain. The theory assumes that there is a direct and in-variant relationship between stimulus intensity and perceived pain. It proposes that undifferentiated free nerve endings are the major, if not the specific, receptors that generate pain impulses. These impulses are carried from the receptors by pain fibers, the small myelinated A-delta fibers and the unmyelinated C fibers, in peripheral nerves to the lateral spinothalamic tract in the spinal cord and then to a pain center in the thalamus (Sweet; Sternbach, 1968; Melzack and Wall, 1970).

There seems to be little question that peripheral and central nervous system pathways have specialized functions related to pain, but there is some doubt that any of these comprise an exclusive pain modality in which there is a fixed stimulus-response relationship. Some opponents of the specificity theory feel that one of its major weaknesses is its psychological assumption. To say that certain receptors and/or fibers respond only to noxious stimulation is a physiological statement. But to say that this stimulation will always be felt as pain is a psychological statement. Stimulation of pain-specific receptors and fibers does not always produce pain, and pain is not the only sensation that may be produced. Many variables affect the transduction properties of receptor-fiber units, such as rate of adaptation and thresholds to mechanical distortion or chemical change. Opponents of this theory suggest that the physiological specialization of nervous system path-ways in the pain mechanism can be accepted as fact without also ac-cepting that stimulation of these pathways will invariably result in feeling pain (Melzack and Wall, 1970).

The specificity theory is helpful in explaining how a person with an intact neurophysiological system perceives and responds to pain when impending or actual tissue damage triggers impulses that travel over the nervous system pathways. In other words, he feels pain because pain pathways have been stimulated. However, when comparable stimuli are applied to several people it does not explain why one person will perceive intense pain, another moderate pain and still another no pain at all. There is not a fixed stimulus-response relationship if tissue damage does not always result in pain. Further, the specificity theory explains why pain may be alleviated after alterations in the pain pathways, such as chordotomy or thalamotomy, but it does not explain why pain may continue or return.

Because of some of the problems encountered in the specificity theory, a pattern theory of the pain mechanism was proposed. The pattern theory actually includes several slightly different theories. All of these theories generally have in common the concept that patterning of the nerve impulses generated by receptors forms the basis of a code that provides the information that there is pain. It is widely accepted that the basis of sensory perceptions is provided by the temporal and spatial patterns of nerve impulses, that is, the patterns associated with the length of time a stimulus lasts and the area it covers. One of the pattern theories stresses a reverberating circuit mechanism (Livingston). Another pattern theory is a specialized input-controlling system (Noordenbos). Still another suggests that the pattern for pain is produced by intense stimulation of nonspecific receptors (Weddell). The latter proposes that all fiber endings are alike, except for those that innervate hair cells. It ignores the evidence that indicates that nervous system pathways have specialized functions related to pain.

The input-control theory suggests that two fiber systems are involved in pain. Normally, the rapidly conducting fiber system inhibits synaptic transmission in the more slowly conducting system that carries the signal for pain. Under pathological conditions the slow system conducting pain establishes dominance over the fast system. The fast system is then unable to inhibit the transmission of pain impulses. This theory explains that pathological pain states result from the central summation of impulses in the slowly conducting fiber system. It also explains that failure to relieve pain by sectioning pain pathways in the spinal cord is due to a "leak" of impulses past the point of sectioning by way of the diffuse connections of the anterolateral pathways. But sectioning of the latter may fail as well.

The reverberating circuit mechanism also relies on central summation and proposes that pathological stimulation sets up reverberating circuits in spinal internuncial pools. These circuits are believed to be closed loops of nerve fibers that stimulate one another in a circular fashion. Once established these circuits can then be triggered by normally non-noxious inputs. This generates the abnormal volleys of nerve impulses up the spinal cord to the brain where they are interpreted as pain. A trigger point may develop in a limb that has been previously injured. The initial injury sets up the reverberating circuit. Then merely touching the limb can stimulate the pools to generate more impulses that would be felt as pain. Even in the absence of touch, the abnormal activity may continue in the circuit. Therefore, pain may continue in the absence of peripheral stimuli. Since at this point the source of pain is actually in the spinal cord itself, it is understandable why some procedures such as neurectomy and sympathectomy do not always alleviate pain. This does not explain, however, why severing pathways in the cord or thalamus may not relieve pain.

More comprehensive than either the specificity theory or the pattern theories is the gate control theory. This theory includes the concepts of physiological specialization and central summation. Basically, it suggests that the small-diameter fibers conduct the excitatory pain signals and that large-diameter cutaneous afferents may inhibit the transmission of pain impulses from the spinal cord to the brain. This is accomplished by a gating mechanism embedded in the cells of the substantia gelatinosa in the dorsal horn of the spinal cord. This gate control mechanism regulates the afferent patterns before they influence the central transmission cells in the dorsal horn. Pain perception and response result when the output of the central transmission cells reaches or exceeds a critical level. In other words, the gating mechanism sums up the net stimulus due to excitatory and inhibitory signals and conveys this net result to the brain. The gate is closed, or pain is prevented, by stimulating large afferent fibers.

The impulses transmitted from the gating mechanism to the central transmission cells are influenced not only by the ratio of activity in large and small fibers but also by brain activities activated by the afferent patterns in the dorsal column system. By way of descending fibers, the brain processes modulate properties of the gate control system. This means that the individual's present and past experiences have an effect on the gate control system. The input is evaluated in terms of its physical properties and meaning to the individual before it is felt as sensation and before it elicits a behavioral response.

The gate control theory explains why comparable stimuli will be felt as pain in one person and not in another because it takes into account the influence of the individual's memory and cognitive processes on the nerve impulses before they are perceived and responded to. It explains why electroanalgesia is often effective in relieving chronic, intractable pain. This method utilizes an electronic-impulse generator percutaneously or surgically implanted to stimulate the inhibitory afferents that close the gate. The theory explains the persistence or return of pain following chordotomy or lobotomy as being due to the longlasting changes, called pain memories in the nervous system, produced by painful stimuli ("Pain," 1970; Melzack, 1970 a and b; Melzack and Wall, 1965, 1970).

Having cited the many neurophysiological processes that could underlie a sensation of pain, it is important to go one step further and examine the mechanism for localization of the pain. This might not be as significant to the nurse or the patient if all pain were felt in an area where a physical stimulus could be identified. Precise localization of pain is thought by some to be due to somatotopic organization in the thalamic nuclei. Others feel it is due to the sensory strip in the sensory cortex, although stimulation of the latter does not produce pain (Elliot; Sternbach, 1968). However, pain is sometimes felt in areas other then those stimulated. This phenomenon is called referred pain and may exist with or without pain at the area of stimulation.

Referred pain.   Referred pain most often occurs with stimulation of deep tissues, especially the viscera. Figures 1 and 2 on the following page illustrate some of the cutaneous areas to which pain in various organs may be referred. This knowledge is helpful to the nurse in explaining to a patient with a common duct stone, for example, that the pain he feels between his shoulders is not necessarily indicative of an additional disease but most likely is referred pain. It is also well to remember that stimulation of the area of referred pain, as well as stimulation of the organ from which the pain is referred, may produce more pain in that area.

There are several theories about the mechanism of referred pain. The convergence theory seems to be the most widely accepted. It proposes that somewhere in the nervous system there is a convergence of nerve impulses from the diseased viscera and from the skin to which the pain is referred. This results in deceptive messages that are then sent to the thalamus and the sensory cortex (Elliott; Melzack and Wall, 1970).

It is well known that it is more difficult for a person to distinguish and locate various sensations in the viscera than it is in the cutaneous tissues. This vague representation of internal sensations occurs even when pain from the viscera is not referred to an area some distance from the viscera. The lack of precision in distinguishing and locating various visceral sensations may be due to the fewer number of receptors in the viscera, lack of experience in localizing these sensations and/or inability to use vision in assisting with localization (Best and Taylor; Sternbach, 1968).

Nursing intervention. Knowledge of the neurophysiological processes underlying the sensation of and response to pain is useful to the nurse in several ways. Some of these have already been suggested in the discussion. Ultimately the nurse's understanding of why the patient feels pain, why the pain is localized in a particular area and why he responds as he does is of great importance in designing nursing intervention. This intervention may range from giving a simple explanation to the patient regarding why he feels pain in the scrotum when he has acute nephritis, to determining measures for pain

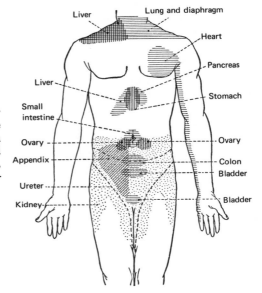

Figure 1. Referred pain, anterior view. This indicates the cutaneous areas to which pain in the various organs is referred (Chaffee and Greisheimer, 1969, p. 269; adapted from Pottenger).

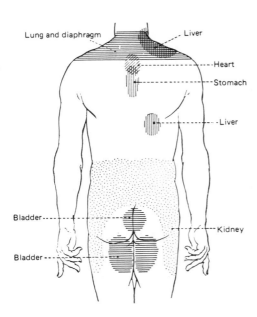

Figure 2. Referred pain, posterior view (Chaffee and Greisheimer, 1969, p. 269; adapted from Pottenger).

alleviation that interrupt the processes underlying the sensation and reaction. Understanding and use of all the theories of the pain mechanism are helpful in planning the most appropriate measures for pain relief. For example, the chronic pain suffered by a patient with metastatic bowel cancer may be explained in several different ways. Each explanation may lead to different methods of intervention, as illustrated in the following. If the patient's pain is explained as stimulation of pain receptors, intervention will include removal of some of the stimulation through appropriate positioning that decreases the amount of pressure exerted by the neoplasm on the bowel. If the pain is explained as intense stimulation of non-specific receptors in the bowel, the nurse may try to diminish the stimulation by eliminating foods in the diet that produce flatus. If pain is explained as dominance of the slowly conducting fiber system that carries the signal for pain, intervention will include attempts to reverse the dominance by the selective use of touch and pressure. Touch and pressure may activate the rapidly conducting fiber system which in turn inhibits the transmission of pain impulses. Or, the pain may be explained as sustained reverberating circuits in the spinal cord that are triggered by normally non-noxious stimuli, and intervention may prevent this by avoiding stimulation of trigger points. If the occurrence of pain is explained as an open gate to the transmission of pain signals because of lack of stimulation to inhibitory signals, the nurse may attempt to close the gate by stimulating the cutaneous afferents with gentle rubbing or vibration.

These are only a few general examples of how the nurse's knowledge of the neurophysiological processes can assist her in arriving at effective intervention. Nursing intervention is most productive when the nurse's assessment includes a detailed account of the pathological condition and the pain mechanisms underlying the patient's pain experience. This involves knowledge of exactly which organs, muscles, nerves and other structures are involved in each patient along with application of each theory of the pain mechanism.

Duration and intensity of pain.   The severity of pain and the length of time it lasts operate together to have a rather distinct effect upon behavioral responses. We have already noted how this influences the physiological responses. Briefly, intense pain may result in activation followed by rebound. If the pain continues, however, adaptation and then stress reaction may occur. We have also seen that some of the theories of the pain mechanism suggest that pain of long duration may establish pain memories in the nervous system or self-sustaining reverberating circuits of pain impulses in the spinal cord that result in the persistence of pain after the noxious stimuli are removed.

Brief pain of low intensity may elicit no observable behavioral response. Conversely, brief pain of high intensity often results in reflex and/or consciously controlled efforts to escape from the cause if this is possible. Touching a hot stove may be followed by a reflex response of withdrawal, and movement that causes muscle spasm may be quickly responded to with rubbing or stretching of the muscle to alleviate the spasm. Brief pain of moderate or high intensity may result in greater acceptance of physical contact for that period of time. Mr. Casey, fifty-two years old, had empyema following pneumonia and experienced unilateral chest pain for over a week. During that time the nurse offered physical contact by touching his hand, but he always removed his hand within a few seconds. However, during a thoracentesis he did accept her touch, and when the needle entered the pleura he squeezed her hand and continued this until the procedure was over.

The patient usually views brief pain of whatever intensity as a more or less isolated event in terms of both his body and the period of time devoted to a response. For example, the pain of a venipuncture or spinal tap is limited to a small area of the body and the behavioral responses for all phases of the pain experience may be relatively brief. After the procedure is over the pain receives little attention; the patient's focus often quickly shifts to other matters. However, if the patient is a child and/or is exposed to multiple episodes of brief pain, each painful occurrence will assume greater significance until their cumulative effect is that of chronic pain. Even a single short episode for a child may evoke intense and long-lasting behavioral responses because of his cognitive level as well as other factors to be discussed later.

Chronic pain is not the isolated event that brief pain is. It is not something that happens to a part of the body. Chronic pain begins to consume the body. It draws all attention to itself and makes it more and more impossible for the patient to attend to anything in the environment that does not seem related to the pain. The patient becomes exhausted. His body movements, verbalizations and vocalizations tend to decrease in intensity and frequency. Moreover, he may begin to wonder why this has happened to him and how it will affect his life. The cultural and psychological factors in the next section come into play as he seeks an answer. During the weeks that Mr. Casey experienced unilateral chest pain he lay in bed almost motionless, usually on his affected side to splint his chest. He rarely initiated conversation. Although he sometimes turned on his television, he frequently failed to turn up the sound to an audible level. Every time he saw his doctor he mentioned that he hoped the doctor would soon find a cure because he needed to get back to work.

Intensity of pain is often reflected in the patient's choice of words to describe his pain, even when he is not asked to rate it by some scale. Slight pain is rarely referred to as pain and the first degrees of pain may even be pleasurable (Keele). Mr. Casey did not describe any pleasurable sensations but there were variations in the terms he used to describe his pain. Upon questioning, he often described the discomfort in his chest as an "ache." But when the intensity increased enough for him to call the nurse to obtain some pain relief measure, he would say his chest "hurt." Following the thoracentesis he used the term "painful" to describe the sensation.

Sometimes patients may feel that intense brief pain or mild chronic pain is easier to endure than the measures required to relieve it. These patients may fail to complain of pain or they may state that the relief measures merely add to the pain or are not worth the trouble. For example, one woman with recurrent breast abscesses stated that the local anesthetic hurt as much as the incision and drainage, and expressed a desire not to receive the local anesthetic. Another woman complained of backache during the last trimester of her pregnancy. The public health nurse helped her with proper body mechanics and demonstrated pelvic rocking, suggesting that this be done for about 15 seconds five or six times a day. On the nurse's next visit the patient said these measures had alleviated the backache. However, on the third visit the patient admitted only upon questioning that her back still hurt, but she said that the exercises were too much trouble.

It is interesting to note that Hardy has found that there is a maximal intensity of pain which can be perceived and that beyond this point an increase in the stimulus will not cause greater pain. But this is small solace to the patient experiencing severe pain.

Alterations in the level of consciousness. The patient's level of consciousness may be lowered or altered due to such factors as head injury, infections of the central nervous system, sedatives, general anesthetics, anticholinergics and conditions that decrease oxygenation of the brain. The patient's responses to pain will vary in accordance with the extent to which the level of consciousness is altered. Of course, the patient who is totally unconscious, regardless of the cause, will not respond to pain or any other stimuli.

Drugs such as scopolamine (an anticholinergic) and phenobarbital (a sedative) depress the central nervous system causing drowsiness and sleep. A different reaction occurs if either of these drugs is administered alone in the presence of pain or in combination with a drug that does not provide adequate pain relief. Either drug may result in restlessness and confusion, and the patient may respond much more vigorously to pain than he would if he were fully conscious. In the aftermath of pain the patient who received phenobarbital may be embarrassed that he had not controlled his behavior in his usual way, whereas with scopolamine the amnesic properties of this drug may cause the patient to forget the pain experience.

One method of obstetric analgesia is a combination of scopolamine and a barbiturate or analgesic. Mrs. Palmer demonstrates the possible effects of these medications. During labor and prior to medication she was awake between contractions, crying quietly for a few seconds and saying that the pain was terrible. She responded to the contractions with muscle tension such as clenched fists and clenched teeth, but she did not verbalize or vocalize. Within an hour after scopolamine and pentobarbital sodium were administered Mrs. Palmer slept between contractions and screamed loudly during the contractions. In the postpartum period she remembered nothing about this part of her labor. If someone had mentioned events that occurred during that time, she probably would have begun to remember.

General anesthetics depress the central nervous system in stages. When they are used for surgery the nurse may observe two stages of recovery from anesthesia in the immediate postoperative period. She may first observe the second stage of anesthesia, the stage of excitement. During this stage the patient may overreact to stimuli expecially noise. The patient then passes into the first stage of anesthesia, often called the stage of analgesia. This implies that the small amount of anesthesia retained in the patient's system provides some pain relief. The patient may awaken and complain of pain, but he is usually drowsy and will fall asleep again. In some diseases such as pneumonia or cerebral arteriosclerosis the oxygen supply to the brain is depleted. Patients with these conditions may also complain of pain and then go to sleep.

Cutaneous versus visceral sites of pain. The site of the painful sensation in terms of whether it is visceral or cutaneous may affect the quality of the sensation, physiological responses, body movement and other behaviors. Cutaneous pain is usually bright and pricking in quality. It tends to elicit fight or flight responses on both the physiological and overt behavioral levels more frequently than does visceral pain. The biological usefulness of the fight or flight reaction has already been suggested with regard to the physiological response of activation. Since external hostile assaults are most likely to pierce the skin first, it is significant that cutaneous pain physiologically prepares the individual to combat or escape the cause of pain (Wolff and Wolf). Besides the physiological changes, the fight or flight responses to cutaneous pain may be observed in angry screams or words. The galvanizing effect of cutaneous pain may be observed in aggressive physical contact. This may include hitting or voluntary and involuntary protective movements such as reflexive withdrawal from the stimulus and shielding the area of pain.

Visceral pain usually has an aching quality and seems to exert a depressing effect on most behavioral responses (Wolff and Wolf). The patient usually remains inactive, a highly appropriate response in view of the virtual impossibility of running away from an attack from within. Although it is not always true, verbal and vocal behaviors tend to be quieter than those accompanying cutaneous pain.

Seven-year-old Charlie demonstrates these different responses. Several hours after a cystoscopy he complained of a "hurt" as he pointed to his lower abdomen where his distended bladder could be easily observed. He remained motionless in bed with a wrinkled forehead and occasionally whined quietly. Earlier that day he had received a subcutaneous injection in preparation for the cystoscopy. During the injection he made repeated attempts to move away from the inserted needle. Throughout the injection of the medication he cried loudly. The distended bladder had a depressing effect upon his responses, the usual effect of visceral pain. The sensation accompanying the injection was more similar to cutaneous pain and elicited flight responses.

Implicit in this discussion of visceral and cutaneous sites of pain is the notion that cutaneous pain is caused by a stimulus external to the body and visceral pain by an internal stimulus. This is usually true due to the location of the skin and viscera. However, responses to pain at these sites may differ according to whether the stimulus is applied from without by a person or a procedure or is applied from within as a result of pathological processes. In fact, the behavioral reaction may be entirely dependent upon whether or not a person or object external to the body can be blamed for the pain regardless of the site or quality of the pain. For example, when the nurse palpated Charlie's bladder, causing further visceral discomfort, he responded by crying loudly and attempting to move away from the nurse. Although the pain was visceral, it was increased by external means and the response resembled that for cutaneous pain.

Environmental conditions.   Solar radiation, extreme cold, wind, high altitudes and air pollution are but a few examples of environmental conditions that may increase pain in persons with various diseases as well as cause pain in healthy individuals.

Exposure to rays from the sun in hot, cold or cloudy weather may cause first, second or even third degree burns. The patient taking regular doses of certain drugs such as chlorpromazine may be photosensitive and develop dermatitis following relatively brief exposure to the sun.

Strong winds may excoriate unprotected areas of skin. A very slight draft may cause severe pain in the patient with second degree burns due to the stimulation of exposed nerve endings. Drafts may also stimulate trigger points of pain.

Extremes in temperature and humidity may also affect some types of pain. Strenuous exercise in hot weather may result in sudden muscle pain (heat cramps) by excessive loss of sodium chloride in perspiration. Very cold weather may cause frostbite, especially in people with poor circulation. It is first felt as numbness, but severe pain may occur as the part is thawed. Patients with musculoskeletal problems such as arthritis tend to experience increased pain in cold weather, particularly following chilling, possibly because the cold results in muscle tension. Many such patients, according to folklore, are able to predict changes in the weather because of increased pain. Underlying this pain may be muscle tension from slight decreases in temperature aggravated by increased humidity since water is a good conductor of temperature and can intensify the cold. These patients often seek a warm, dry climate. Low humidity may increase the irritation of an inflamed respiratory tract. Some patients find that warm air increases efforts to breathe and thereby increases discomfort.

Low pressures of oxygen may result in pain in a healthy person as well as in patients with pathological processes that already endanger the oxygen supply. At high altitudes the percentage of oxygen is actually the same as it is at sea level; however, since the barometric pressure is reduced at these altitudes, the partial pressure of oxygen is also diminished. Consequently there may be inadequate delivery of oxygen to tissues depending, of course, upon the altitude and the rate of ascent (Winton and Bayliss). Since the cabins in commercial airlines are pressurized, flight does not ordinarily present a problem. But rapid ascent into the mountains by car, for example, may precipitate a crisis in the patient with sickle-cell anemia or cause migraine headache in a person with a history of vascular headaches. The patient with peripheral vascular disease is rarely affected by rapid ascent to high altitudes. But a patient with arterosclerotic heart disease may experience anginal pain if he exerts himself at high altitudes. In the healthy person the phenomenon of "mountain sickness" may occur with headache and other symptoms. In addition to the effects of low oxygen pressure, the low barometric pressure at high altitudes may cause abdominal pain from distension of the organs. Or, patients with chronic lung disease may experience increased chest pain because of the difficulty in expelling mucous. Coughing is less effective in dislodging particles and the respiratory tract is irritated even in the healthy individual.

Air pollution, which promises to become an increasing problem, may be another cause of pain. Large particulate pollution such as sand may cause minor irritation of the eyes. But a greater problem results from irritant gases such as oxides of nitrogen, sulfur gas, sulfate and ozones. These chemicals are thought to combine with water at the tissue level in the lungs, eyes, nose and other areas, producing acids that irritate the tissues and cause pain. The resulting inflammation may be only mildly uncomfortable for the healthy individual, but it may be severely painful or fatal to the patient with chronic lung disease.

Sensory restriction.   This concept refers to an external environment that does not contain stimuli adequate to maintain the individual's optimal level of cortical arousal. The stimuli may be inadequate in amount, patterning or variation. This results in numerous observable behaviors that reflect changes in physiological functioning, learning, cognition, perception, motor ability and affect. Among these effects of sensory restriction is an increased sensitivity to painful stimuli, a decreased tolerance for pain and an increase in the number of mild discomforts.

Three types of sensory restriction have been researched and any of them may occur in patient settings in or out of the hospital. Each one may exist for any or all sensory modalities. One is sensory deprivation, defined as the lowest possible reduction of stimuli. An example is visual sensory deprivation in the form of bilateral eye patches. The patient may be able to perceive some visual input but it is reduced to as low a level as possible. A second type of sensory restriction is perceptual deprivation, defined as reduction in the patterning and meaningful organization of sensory input. A patient in an intensive care unit may experience auditory perceptual deprivation because of the overriding sounds of cardiac monitors, suction machines, oxygen equipment and the like. The third type is perceptual monotony, defined as a lack of variation in stimuli. The stimuli are received at an adequate level and are understandable to the patient, but repetitive. This situation frequently occurs with the patient confined to his bed or his home. It usually involves the senses of hearing, sight, touch, and sometimes smell and taste.

The human being is motivated to obtain sensory input sufficient to maintain an optimum level of cortical arousal. When the environment is inadequate, centrally regulated thresholds for sensation tend to be lowered, allowing the person to utilize more of the available input. Consequently, sensitivity to pain, as well as tactile, visual and auditory stimuli, may be greater. In other words, under conditions of sensory restriction the patient will probable react to pain of lesser intensity than that required for a reaction under conditions of adequate input (Schultz). It is a common observation that pain seems to be more severe at night, and this is probably due in part to perceptual monotony. Frequently, the patient is alone in a quiet room with only the unvarying input from his four walls and his bed. In addition to the seemingly greater intensity of pain, the patient is usually less able to tolerate pain. During the day when there is a greater amount and variation of sensory input, the patient may not request pain relief measures for a certain intensity of pain. But at night he may find the same intensity of pain unbearable.

A patient who previously did not experience pain may begin to complain of various aches and discomforts when he is subjected to sensory restriction. Research on groups of 15 to 100 men confined together for several months in the limited area of a military base in the Antarctic (perceptual monotony) showed a progressive increase in somatic complaints such as soreness of muscles, upset stomach, headaches and chest pain (Schultz). Mrs. Farrell demonstrated some of this during her eight weeks of hospitalization for a series of grafts to her burned arm. She had no visitors, since her home was several hundred miles away. After a few weeks she received very few cards and letters. The physician had ordered 10 grains of acetylsalicylic acid p.r.n. Mrs. Farrell requested this mostly for "a little bit of a headache" and an "ache all over." She never asked for this medication on days when she was able to find a patient who would play cards with her.

Physical strain and fatigue. This aspect of the physical and physiological factors that affect pain sensation and response covers a wide variety of conditions. The following discussion will focus on temporary mechanical strain on body parts and on fatigue resulting from inadequate sleep and rest.

One of the most difficult types of pain to control is the brief but intense pain felt during the first 24 to 48 hours postoperatively when the patient attempts to move the structures involved in the surgery. Certain body positions and movements may place substantial mechanical strain on the operative area such as pulling on the sutures and contraction or spasm of cut muscles. Other examples of physical strain are weightbearing on inflamed joints and exercise of contracted muscles. These types of mechanical pull or pressure on a painful area may increase the sensation of pain. Consequently the patient typically attempts to avoid positions and movements that increase the strain.

Repeated physical strain, whether or not it increases pain, or inadequate rest and sleep may lead to physical fatigue. Fatigue from lack of sleep results in symptoms that may affect the patient's behavioral response to pain. (The overall effects are remarkably similar to those of sensory restriction.) Quite understandably the feelings of tiredness and weariness cause the individual to begin to take the easy way out, choosing alternatives that demand the least of him physically and mentally. Since fatigue delays transmission of nerve impulses, reaction times may become uneven. As the mental processes slow down it becomes difficult to maintain a train of thought. Fantasies become more prevalent and hallucinations may occur. An excellent example of this is the experience of a disc jockey who stayed awake to broadcast for over eight days. On the last morning of this marathon, during one of the routine medical examinations, he decided the physician was an undertaker who had come to bury him, and immediately ran out of the building (Current Research on Sleep and Dreams, 1965).

Such effects of sleep deprivation suggest that fatigue will affect the patient's response to pain in several ways. He will have less energy and mental ability to utilize his usual strategies such as distraction or imagination for coping with pain. As a result he will tend to choose less demanding alternatives such as analgesics. In addition he may indulge in horrible fantasies about the significance of his pain. This in turn may increase the subjective experience of the pain sensation. One example of some of these effects is a maternity patient who refused analgesics and anesthetics until she had labored for 24 hours and had been without sleep for 36 hours. At that point she began to say that the labor would never end and that her baby would die. A half hour later she accepted an epidural block.

How do cultural influences affect the patient's behavioral responses to pain and the pain sensation?

The culture in which a patient lives for the greater part of his life has a tremendous influence upon his attitudes toward pain and his manifestations of suffering. In this time a person learns what the members of his culture expect and accept with regard to painful experiences. The cultural expectations may be very detailed, specifying such things as: different reaction patterns according to sex, age and occupation; whether curative or palliative treatment should be sought; the intensity and duration of pain that should be tolerated; what responses should be made; to whom pain should be reported; and what types of pain require attention. It is this latter aspect of cultural prescription that may influence the pain sensation itself. For example, a cut or bruise obtained under conditions such as participation in a sport may be an expected and accepted consequence, and the victim may perceive the pain as being of lesser intensity than he would if a comparable injury occurred in a situation where it was not expected. However, it is probably more common that the *perceived* intensity of pain is unchanged, but that pain *tolerance* is affected.

One mechanism that assists in understanding how cultural expectations are learned is operant conditioning. This procedure is based on the principle that behaviors followed by reward tend to occur more frequently, and that those followed by punishment or lack of attention tend to be extinguished. Beginning in childhood, certain behavioral responses to pain are rewarded and others are punished or ignored. In one culture the child's crying response to pain may be followed by cuddling and sympathy from the parent. In another, the crying may be ignored and the parent may matter-of-factly care for the injury, praising the child when he stops crying. With each painful experience the child learns more of the nuances of acceptable attitudes toward pain and responses to pain. By the time he reaches adulthood these may be very firmly established reactions.

Considering the effectiveness of current mass communications media and the ease with which a person can travel or change his place of residence, it is not surprising that there is an increasing number of variations within each culture. Even in adulthood this exposure to the expectations of other cultures and subcultures may result in some change in the person's behavioral responses to the pain experience, although the underlying attitudes may change more slowly. Therefore, it is wise for the nurse to avoid stereotyping a patient's behavioral response to pain on the basis of her knowledge of the expectations of his culture. Knowledge of different cultural traditions is more helpful to the nurse in other ways.

First of all, the nurse learns that there are ways of responding to pain other than her own. Although some of these may be frowned upon in her culture, they may be not only accepted but very desirable in the patient's culture. This knowledge helps the nurse understand and appreciate the many different behaviors she may see, and it assists her in discounting her own cultural traditions as a means of assessing the patient's pain experience. Hopefully, this will prevent the nurse from avoiding and punishing the patient who behaves in a manner that is unacceptable in her own culture. In addition, she will know that the presence or absence of expressions such as crying and moaning do not necessarily indicate the same pain experience in people of different cultural backgrounds. For example, mild pain may elicit crying in one patient. Another may never cry regardless of the intensity or implications of the pain and a third may cry only with intense pain.

Secondly, knowledge of the various cultural attitudes toward pain assists the nurse in determining the significance of pain to the patient. Her intervention will be more effective when she seeks such clues as those that indicate whether the pain is viewed as punishment or identification with God, whether the patient seeks immediate relief or a cure for the pain, and whether the patient both expects and accepts pain or merely expects but cannot accept pain.

The following discussion will focus on variations in attitudes toward pain and responses to pain which are due to the different cultural expectations resulting from the patient's sociocultural background, his sex, age and religion, the body part involved in the pain, and the roles ascribed to members of the health team.

Membership in a particular sociocultural group. It would be impossible to cover all the expectations of the various cultural groups the nurse may encounter. Therefore a few cultural groups have been selected to demonstrate some of the differences in cultural traditions. These are "Old Americans," Italians, Jews and Irish, based on Zborowski's (1952, 1969) systematic study, and the Southern Negroes and other deprived minority groups. When the nurse cares for a patient from some other cultural group, the differences exemplified here may serve as a guide to her observations and readings regarding that group's expectations.

The "Old American" group as defined in Zborowski's study, includes all ages of adulthood. Its members are typically born in the United States, white, Protestant and without identification with any foreign group either nationally or socially. The cultural expectations of this group are dominant in the United States; most nurses reading this book will possess the attitudes and behaviors common to it. The Old American usually attempts to give an efficient description of his pain to members of the health profession; otherwise he remains nonexpressive. He attempts to control reflexive responses of withdrawal and to avoid screaming, crying and other manifestations of pain. He views such vocalizations as useless and indicative of a defeated condition. Only limited expressions such as an occasional jerk or "ouch" are acceptable. He takes pride in being the "good patient" who does not annoy others with his complaints. In the presence of family and friends he tries to retain his sense of humor, to minimize his pain and not to evoke sympathy or pity. When the pain becomes severe he tends to withdraw and wants to be alone. He is optimistically future-oriented, concerned with the implications of his pain but confident that skillful health team members will effect a cure. In the meantime, however, he feels that the pain is unnecessary and expects it to be relieved by palliative measures. Before this patient seeks medical assistance, he may experience some anxiety and conflict in deciding whether his pain is insignificent or is a warning signal that something is wrong with his body. He does not want to ignore a warning signal but on the other hand he does not want to feel he is a "sissy." Pain involved in athletic performance is expected but not accepted; however, such pains as headaches, "growing pains" in the extremities, stomachaches and sore throats are accepted as normal unless they increase in frequency and severity. With any pain the patient may delay contacting the physician a few days to see if it goes away.

The patient of the Jewish religion has a low tolerance for pain and tends to give rather dramatic accounts of his pain experience. He uses many adjectives such as "terrific" and "unbearable." He does not mind telling others about his more extreme responses to it. Although this behavior differs markedly from the Old American response, the Old American and the Jew share a similar attitude toward pain. They are both future-oriented and concerned with the symptomatic significance of the pain. The Jew, however, is pessimistic, especially at first, and his reactions initially tend to be more intense, apparently for the purpose of creating sufficient concern to cause others to take the best possible care of him. Unlike the Old American, he believes that crying and moaning help by mobilizing those around him to offer sympathy and assistance. He does not want to be alone with his pain. Another source of his pessimism is that he does not view the physician as an undisputable authority. He may seek the advice of several physicians. But he is not afraid of the diagnosis since it is usually less ominous than what he had imagined. Because the Jew is primarily concerned about the future implications of pain and in spite of his low tolerance for pain, he seeks curative measures and frequently is reluctant to take analgesics, expecially if they are addicting.

The Italian, like the Jew, has a low tolerance for pain and feels that it is natural to cry, moan, complain and use many gestures and body movements. This response apparently serves no particular purpose such as mobilization of support—it is merely natural. Unlike the Jew he does not complain to his family for fear that he will upset them. Besides, he feels that they know of his pain without being told and that they want to help. He likes to have family and friends around (if they do not remind him of his pain by asking questions) because their presence tends to take his mind off the pain. In fact he feels he can deal better with the pain if he remains occupied to the extent of going to work. Unlike the Jew, the Italian is present-oriented. The Italian is concerned with the pain sensation itself and not the reasons for the pain. Like the Old American he wants at least palliative relief and he wants it immediately. He believes he should ask for relief as soon as pain occurs. He willingly accepts almost any pain relief measure although he tends to view drugs as unnatural. Interestingly enough, the Italian is among the very few who feel that drugs relieve pain mostly through their psychological effect. In general he has confidence in the health team and complies with their instructions. Surgery is accepted if it relieves pain and does not reduce life's enjoyments (a chordotomy may be refused since it affects sexual functioning). To the Italian the significance of pain is related to its effect upon his state of mind. He experiences depression over the loss of energy and ability to enjoy life. His tears are not only an expression of pain but also a manifestation of grief. Relief of pain immediately relieves the depression.

The Irishman is similar to the Old American in his calm and unemotional reaction to pain. He too feels that complaining serves no purpose. He is reluctant to discuss his pain and suffering. Also like the Old American, the Irishman tends to withdraw from family and friends when he is in pain. However, underlying the Irishman's behavioral responses to pain is an attitude quite different from the Old American. The Old American wants to be alone because he does not want to be seen as weak and helpless, but the Irishman does not mind admitting to his friends that he suffers—he merely wants to suffer alone. He is not expected to share any of his troubles with anyone. It is even difficult to obtain information regarding the quality and intensity of his pain. Whereas the Old American has a low tolerance for pain in that he feels pain is unnecessary and should be relieved, the Irishman seems almost proud of being able to handle pain. His two predominant methods of dealing with pain are relaxing and fighting. To use the passive technique of relaxing the patient must be undisturbed and alone to concentrate on absorbing the pain without complaint. Fighting, an active response, requires mobilizing his resources, "hanging on" and gritting his teeth or continuing to be active by going to work. Often he goes through a long period of struggling with his pain before he consults a physician. When the Irishman finally goes to the physician, he tends to follow orders without question in spite of some skepticism. Perhaps because he has the techniques of relaxing or fighting to assist him, the Irishman is less concerned with the sensation of pain than he is with its future implications. This concern is not focused on the pathological aspects but on possible crippling and inactivity. The patient has less anxiety about this if the pain is caused by external injury such as a fall. Pains resulting from violent sport and fist fights are both expected and accepted without complaint.

The Southern Negro's behavioral response to pain, as reported by McCabe, includes identification of pain in general terms, hesitation to ask for pain relief and sometimes denial of pain when there were sound reasons for suspecting its existence. Since Chapman found a low threshold for reaction to pain in the Negro, it seems probable that in many instances of denial the patient was actually experiencing pain. The purposes and attitudes underlying the Southern Negro's response to pain are not well known. This author (McCaffery) speculates that the patient is distrustful of the care he receives from the predominantly white health team members and that he is attempting to win their favor by simulating the responses of which he knows they approve. The author's personal experience suggests that the Southern Negro does not seek medical assistance until his condition approaches an emergency state. Once he enters the hospital he experiences a quiet panic over his conflict between wanting help and distrusting it. As a result he may leave the hospital against medical advice. More often he stays and tends to respond to care with unquestioning submission, asking for no information and no help. This patient's failure to complain may well be a result of the continuing conflict between need and distrust, for he may feel that if he fails to report symptoms he will be subjected to less of the care he distrusts.

It seems likely that any member of a minority group that is deprived educationally, economically and occupationally as is the Southern Negro may respond in some of the same ways. If his daily life is controlled by a dominant group and if existence is a day-to-day struggle, he can hardly be expected to trust members of the dominant group. Of necessity he has a more present-oriented attitude. He may attempt to behave in a manner approved of by the dominant group since, as Zborowski (1969) found with the Italian, for example, he knows expressive behavior annoys the Old American.

The pain-associated attitudes and behaviors of the Old American, the Jew, the Italian, the Irishman and the Southern Negro demonstrate the wide variations to which the nurse may be exposed. They were not presented for the purpose of telling the nurse what to expect of and how to understand a patient who is a member of one of these cultural groups; too many variations exist for this to be possible. This information may be useful to the nurse in other ways, as the following summary indicates.

First, it becomes obvious that the pain sensation itself probably does not influence the patient's attitude and behavioral responses as much as the patient's cultural background. The nurse must realize that his responses are very effective methods of communicating with members of his culture who will disapprove if he fails to respond according to their traditions.

Secondly, the difference between groups indicates why members of one cultural group often have difficulty understanding the attitudes and responses of members of another. Typically, the Old American is annoyed with the expressions of the Jew and the Italian. The Italian thinks it rather funny that the Jew and Old American are so concerned with the future. In turn the Jew and Old American believe the Italian's behavior is childish and immature. The Italian and Jew think the Old American is rather coldblooded and selfish in not communicating his pain experience. Each considers his own attitudes and behavior the correct ones. The nurse must know that the patient responds in a certain way because he has been taught that this is correct and normal. If she considers that the expectations of her own culture are the only correct and normal ones, she may be prone to make the errors cited by Zborowski (1969). He found that patients with expressive and emotional responses to pain were labeled "mental cases" and sometimes were transferred to psychiatric wards. The nurse from the Old American culture should realize that if she were hospitalized in Italy her failure to express her pain emotionally might result in her being labeled masochistic.

Thirdly, and most importantly, this survey of some cultural expectations regarding pain points out several questions the nurse must ask about her patients. Since similar responses to pain do not necessarily reflect similar attitudes toward it, and since many variations may exist between and within cultural groups, answers to these questions are very pertinent. Is the patient concerned about the pain sensation itself or about the future implications of the pain? Is he afraid the pain indicates fatal illness, or is he afraid the pain does or will deprive him of some specific pleasures of life? Does the patient want to be asked about his pain, or would he rather not be reminded of it? Does he want to be alone for fear of showing an emotional response to pain, or does he want to be alone because he has methods of handling the pain by himself? Does he want visitors to share his pain or does he want to use them as a distraction? Does he expect to obtain pain relief immediately or does he expect he should suffer for a while? Does it matter to him whether he receives palliative or curative pain relief? Does he want to know his diagnosis or is he unconcerned or afraid of it? Does he believe drugs are unnatural pain-relief measures or does he fear the consequences of taking addictive drugs? Does he have confidence in the health team or is he distrustful of their actions or skeptical of their skill? Does his crying mean he wants immediate pain relief, sympathy or demonstration of technical skill? Does he view his expressions of pain as natural, serving a particular purpose, or indicative of defeat?

Age and Sex. The patient's age and sex often determine the acceptability of certain deviations from the norm of his cultural group. In most cultures the female child is allowed greater freedom in the expression of pain then are any other members. In the United States, where the Old American cultural traditions are dominant, young boys are taught at an early age to be brave and not to cry when they hurt themselves. One example of this effect occurred with Bob, 20 months old, white and from a rural area in the mountains of Tennessee. During his hospitalization a cut-down for intravenous fluid was performed. At the beginning of the procedure, as the local anesthetic was being injected, he looked up at his mother standing beside his crib. He was clenching his teeth and tears were forming in his squinted eyes. After a few seconds his mother told him it would be all right to cry, and he did so loudly (McCaffery, 1969).

In general the adult woman is allowed more emotional expression of pain than the man. The man is allowed more freedom as he grows older. For example, an Irishman, who considered himself old, readily admitted to moaning and groaning, which would be unacceptable in a younger man. Any older man not only is more prone to show his pain, but delays longer in consulting a physician and tends to value the physician's personality more than his skill (Zborowski, 1969).

Religion. In most cultural groups one religion is dominant such as the Protestant faith in the Old American. But there are many variations of each religion characterized, for example, as orthodox, reformed, liberal or fundamental. Within each cultural group a member's response to pain may differ slightly because of his particular religious affiliation. The patient's religious faith may serve as a source of either strength or despair. One patient may effectively use prayer and religious ritual to help him tolerate his pain; another may feel that pain is a punishment for his sins and may pray for forgiveness. Miss Berry, 73 years old and of the Southern Baptist denomination, experienced pain from pathological fractures and prayed loudly for forgiveness when the pain became intense. In her prayers she frequently asked God what she had done to deserve such pain. On the other hand, when pain is viewed as punishment it may relieve the patient's guilt feelings. He may therefore endure the pain with a patience and tranquility not present during health. Still another patient may see pain as a means of identifying with God, or he may feel that God has a reason for providing him with an experience of pain.

It is important to note that the association of pain with punishment may occur for reasons other than the patient's religion. The infliction of pain is one of the oldest forms of punishment; therefore, it is not surprising that pain and punishment may be closely related in the patient's mind. A child may consciously associate the pain of illness and treatment with punishment. In the adult this association is likely to be on a more unconscious level.

Body part involved in pain. In almost every culture the members are taught that certain parts of the body are socially unacceptable for viewing and as topics of conversation. Consequently, when pain strikes these areas of the body, the patient's response will differ from his response to pain in an acceptable and acknowledged part of the body. For example, in the United States pain occurring in the genitalia, rectum or anus does not evoke much sympathy from others and is rarely discussed, so the patient may hesitate to complain of the pain. Further, he may find it difficult to describe because he has not been allowed to use such terminology. He may also avoid any protective or rubbing body movements that could indicate the site of pain. Mr. Call, 40 years old, was admitted for urological examinations because of persistent cystitis. The physician ordered Pyridium orally q6h p.r.n. for burning on urination, but Mr. Call rarely requested the medication. Most of the time he received it only when the physician, following his visit with the patient, asked the nurse to give it. Often Mr. Call would turn his head away when a nurse asked him if he had any burning. Apparently this patient was somewhat uncomfortable in making any reference to pain in his genitalia.

Roles ascribed to members of the health team. In the section that discussed membership in a particular sociocultural group, mention was made of differing attitudes toward the physician and the health team in general. In addition to the patient's attitude of confidence or skepticism and the value he places on skill or personality, the patient may inaccurately ascribe various activities to members of the health team according to their occupational titles, age or sex.

He may believe that the physician's role is broader and the nurse's narrower than is actually the case. For example, he may not believe that the nurse is competent to explain or relieve pain. If the nurse suggests that a change in position may relieve his pain, the patient may not do so until his physician suggests it. On the other hand, the patient may think that the nurse, the aide and the physician all have comparable abilities to diagnose and treat pain.

Sometimes the sex of the physician or nurse influences the patient's confidence; also, the age of the health team member may be important. For example, Mr. Call, mentioned in the previous section, requested his Pyridium only from the older nurses and often asked them if they thought he should take it. In addition to his hesitancy in complaining of pain in the genitalia, Mr. Call also seemed more trusting of the knowledge of his male physician and the older female nurses.

What are the psychological factors influencing the patient's behavior and the pain sensation?

Psychological factors account for many variations between members of a particular sociocultural group. Although these occur within the context of the expectations transmitted by members of the cultural group, they can be differentiated from cultural influences on the basis of being the patient's combined interpretation of cultural traditions and his own unique life experience.

Some of the psychological factors to be discussed here are mostly a product of the immediate situation. These include: the degree of powerlessness experienced by the patient; the presence and attitudes of other people; the amount of information given the patient; the degree of threat the pain imposes on his life situation; and the perceptual dominance of pain. Other psychological factors are: his own personal past experience with pain; his cognitive level; the extent to which he has used pain for secondary gains; and his basic algesic type. All the above psychological factors are capable of influencing his expectations of pain, his behavioral response to pain and the actual sensation of pain.

Emotionally traumatic life experiences. Pains that appear to originate solely from the person's psychological or mental state were described in Chapter 1 and included hysterical and hypochondriacal pain. These seem to result from repeated and severe difficulties with emotional problems such as inability to establish meaningful relationships with others or guilt feelings over the conflict between love and aggression. Other painful conditions such as peptic ulcer and ulcerative colitis may be initiated or sustained by various emotional conflicts, but the painful sensation can usually be related to tissue damage. The pain sensation experienced by a person with these psychological problems seems either to be created for the purpose of dealing with the anxiety and guilt, or to be a natural and unavoidable consequence of the physiological effects of anxiety and depression. Unfortunately, pain or illness may be the most effective way the person can cope with his emotional problems. The patient with hysterical pain, for example, is notably free of anxiety. Premature translation of the meaning of his painful symptom may relieve the pain but cause severe anxiety.

The creation or result of pain in handling psychological problems apparently arises from emotionally traumatic life experiences. However, such experiences are generally felt to be frequently recurring events in the patient's past rather than a single traumatic situation in either the past or present. The latter may, however, precipitate the onset of pain. Mrs. Hodges, 47 years old, is a good example of this. She was admitted for chest pain of undetermined origin. Her medical history was incredibly long and confusing, involving countless illnesses with unconfirmed diagnoses, contacts with numerous physicians and approximately 15 hospitalizations. She was very willing to talk with the nurse about her past medical problems. Although her factual accounts were often vague and somewhat contradictory, one theme was outstanding—her symptoms and illnesses were almost always associated with the loss of someone she loved. Sometimes a loved one merely moved out of her home and other times a husband (she had been married several times) or relative died. The day before the onset of this episode of chest pain, her niece and the niece's child, who had lived with Mrs. Hodges for several months, had left the state to join the niece's husband.

An emotionally traumatic situation may result in pain in persons who have not been subjected to the sort of life experiences that result in psychological pathology. Many situations in life realistically cause a person to feel depressed, anxious, guilty or frightened. The person may be unable to complain about this personal unhappiness and may project his emotion onto the accompanying physiological effects of his emotion. Thus, he may complain of a stomachache or a headache. This happens in both children and adults. One study of children between four and 14 years of age, who had had more than one episode of abdominal pain, found that most of the children could associate their pain with fear and anxiety. Many of the fears were about the home situation (Lambert). Simply stated, personal unhappiness may be expressed as a painful sensation. It is perhaps easier for the person to talk about the pain than the unhappiness.

Secondary gains of the patient's complaint of pain. Usually the primary gain or reward for complaining of pain is obtaining pain relief through either palliative or curative means. Of equal or more importance, however, may be the other outcomes. The patient may find that complaints of pain elicit sympathy, prevent loneliness, enable him to control the actions of others, allow him to be dependent upon others and avoid certain responsibilities, or prevent others from criticizing him. If any of these are important goals to him that he has been unable to achieve in other ways, they act as significant external rewards for complaints of pain and thereby increase the tendency to complain further (based on the principles of operant conditioning). The complaints may be obvious or subtle and may be persistent. They may be voiced to health team members and the patient's family and friends. This usage of pain appears to be in part a product of childhood development. The crying infant receives the care of his mother and complaints of pain then become powerful help-seeking symbols.

The use of pain complaints for secondary gains may be almost inseparable from the painful conditions created by or associated with emotionally traumatic life experiences. In these instances pain may result in the external rewards mentioned above as well as the internal rewards of avoiding the original anxiety or depression. The patient is able to ignore feelings of fear or loss by focusing his attention on the painful symptom, waiting for it and treating it. Pain can become his major object of interest and the most important thing in his life. Mrs. Hodges, discussed in the previous section, appeared to have pain as a result of personal losses. She seemed to attend to the pain, not the loss. Further, she was able to obtain secondary gain from her pain complaints. Mere mention of chest pain originally brought a nurse and sometimes a physician to her bedside, resulting in a decrease in her feelings of loneliness.

Personal past experience with pain. The importance of the patient's own past experience with pain should not be underestimated and probable cannot be overestimated. Whether or not he has experienced pain, the number of times he has had pain and the associated circumstances will determine whether or not he is conditioned to expect pain, feel a pain sensation and endure pain. This is called classical conditioning in which two stimuli are paired, the conditioned and unconditioned one. For example, Pavlov (1927) found that alarm or defense reactions could be initiated by any stimulus that had been previously associated with injuries, dangerous threat situations or frustrations. Dogs were conditioned to experience a pain response at the mere sight of the symbol for infliction of pain. Clearly, once pain has been experienced, psychic stimuli are capable of triggering the mechanism for pain in the absence of peripheral stimulation. This is illustrated by Mr.

Armstrong, 24 years old, who received the wrong anesthetic for an appendectomy. The surgery was cancelled and he was taken to the recovery room. Upon awakening he complained of abdominal pain. He may have been conditioned to experience pain on the basis of his past experiences or as a result of his knowledge or observations.

The patient may also be conditioned to receive pain relief from various treatments. Almost every nurse has had the experience of giving an injection of an analgesic and having the patient report pain relief almost immediately afterwards, many minutes before the medication could possible have been absorbed. One explanation for this is that the patient has experienced pain relief after an injection of an analgesic often enough to become conditioned. Pain relief has been paired with the process of the injection itself and the injection alone becomes the stimulus for pain relief. This may explain why placebos work.

The patient's experiences with pain do not necessarily result in responses as firmly established as conditioned ones. For example, David, 11 years old, was about to receive a preanesthetic injection and acknowledged that he thought it would hurt. The nurse asked when and what was his last injection. He said it was penicillin about a year ago. She told him this injection would not hurt as much, and David then proceeded to get into position for the injection. After it was over he told the nurse she was correct. It is interesting to speculate whether or not he would have found the present injection as painful as the penicillin if the nurse had not introduced additional information.

Past painful experiences, therefore, may condition pain responses or may be utilized by the patient to determine what might happen to him in another similar situation. In addition, numerous experiences with pain during childhood appear to have a rather generalized effect on the patient's response as an adult. The fact that lower socioeconomic level is a frequent correlate of increased pain sensitivity has been interpreted as meaning that increased experience with pain during childhood results in increased pain sensitivity in adulthood. It is likely that children from the lower socioeconomic levels have more painful experiences than children from higher socioeconomic levels. Therefore, those adults who had greater experience with pain in childhood are most likely to perceive pain as threatening and to be more sensitive to painful stimuli (Collins).

Upon first consideration of the effects of past painful experiences upon the patient's behavior and attitude, it is tempting to believe that the more experience a patient has the more "used to it" he will be. It would seem that he would be less sensitive to pain and less threatened by it. While this may be true for some patients, the bulk of the evidence suggests that it is generally untrue.

Knowledge, understanding and cognitive level. This section refers to the extent to which a patient is able to obtain accurate information and then organize and process it to achieve an understanding of his pain experience. Nursing assessment should include asking the patient what he has been told about the anticipation and experience of pain, who told him, whether or not he believes it, whether or not it contradicts other information or his own experience, and what he believes will relieve his pain. Finding out from others what they have told the patient is useful only to the extent that it enables the nurse to assess the patient's ability to retain and understand what he is told. It is a mistake to assume that a patient possesses information simply because someone has told him. With young children who lack facility with language the nurse's assessment must include observations of other behavioral responses to events, equipment and people.

How much a person believes or knows about the cause, implication and duration of his pain will influence his response to pain and perhaps even its intensity and existence. It is not uncommon for a patient to have unquestioning beliefs or preconceived ideas about pain. The adult patient may utilize what friends have told him or what he has read or seen. Anyone who has ever mentioned his illness to others is familiar with the wealth of free information and advice he is likely to receive from well-meaning friends and relatives.

One patient called for the nurse in a panic to report that he was having a heart attack. In actuality he was experiencing referred chest pain from abdominal distention. Nevertheless this patient refused to ambulate until the physician arrived and listened to his heart. He later commented that a friend of his had had a heart attack and had warned him to be alert for chest pain.

In addition, the layman in this country is informed about diseases through the mass media. Some information may be accurate and helpful while some is devastatingly wrong.

Lack of information can also have a detrimental effect upon the patient's pain experience. For example, Mrs. Jones had a regional anesthetic for excision of a growth on her foot. During the surgery she suddenly screamed, "I can feel it! Stop! It hurts!" After the patient had been calmed, the nurse discovered that pressure, which the patient could feel, had been misinterpreted as pain. The patient had not been told that pressure might be felt.

Incomplete or inaccurate information not only influences the meaning of a painful sensation and the existence of a painful sensation, but also affects the level of anxiety during the period of anticipation of pain. Conditions that promote anxiety and fear of pain tend to result in overestimation of the intensity of the painful stimuli. In general, the more severe the anxiety the greater the reaction to pain stimulation

(Bronzo and Powers; Jones, Bentler and Petry; Malmo and Shagass).

There are two categories of information that appear to be especially relevant to the amount of anxiety experienced during the anticipation of pain. One is when the pain will be felt. When the patient does not know how long he will have to wait before the painful sensation is felt, his anxiety tends to increase. For example, if a patient is told he will have a spinal tap "sometime today" he is likely to be much more anxious than if he is told that the spinal tap will be done at ten o'clock that morning. It is also probable that the longer the period of anticipation the higher the anxiety, unless this period of time is used to reduce anxiety. The second type of information concerns the intensity and duration of pain and the harmful effects that may be associated with it. Anxiety tends to be particularly high when the patient anticipates that some of the pain he will feel may be indicative of harmful effects that are beyond the control of the physician. For example, if the patient believes that some of the pain associated with the spinal tap may mean that the physician has hit a nerve that will result in long-lasting or permanent back pain, his anxiety will increase. He will tend to overestimate the intensity of the pain and be less tolerant of it. Also, if the patient is not told approximately how long the painful sensation will last, he may have a vague notion that the pain will last indefinitely or that once it subsides it could return at any time. Of course, this increases anxiety and heightens pain responses. The patient's anxiety is also increased if he anticipates that the pain will be severe. If the pain is of lesser intensity he is still likely to evaluate it at a higher intensity or to be less tolerant of it since he expects it to become worse.

Many patients remark that it is easier to endure the pain itself than it is to wait for it, not knowing what it will be like or when it will occur. Clearly, the period of anticipation of pain is a time when uncertainty may cause a great increase in anxiety. And when the pain occurs, this high level of anxiety tends to result in an overestimation of the intensity of the pain.

The patient's information about pain may include ideas about pain relief. He may have been told by a friend that "shots are the only way" to get pain relief. Or he may favor a home remedy handed down from one generation to another. A television commercial may have convinced him that a particular product is the most effective. For example, Jane, 11 years old, voiced her belief about pain remedies when she requested Alka-Seltzer for her headache associated with a possible brain tumor.

The young child cannot rely as heavily as the adult on verbal and written information. He uses his observations of the pain responses of others and the type of equipment used in painful procedures as one source of information about pain. If a child sees another child cry with pain when the physician examines him, the observing child may ask,

"Is the doctor going to do that to me?" The child also tends to anticipate pain on the basis of the equipment associated with it. Syringes and shining steel objects are frequently used in painful procedures. The child may anticipate pain whenever he sees such instruments. Merely being approached by a nurse or physician may cause him to fear pain.

Cognitive ability.   Of course, regardless of the number of accurate facts a child or adult may have about pain, he may still be unable to be logical about them due to his level of cognitive functioning. Cognitive ability, mentioned in Chapter 2, involves the extent to which a person organizes what he knows. It is well to remember that a person may possess a great deal of information without being able to see relationships between various aspects and without being able to organize it into a coherent whole. For example, the nurse talked with Mr. Stewart about his gastric pain and he explained that he knew this was caused by "too much acid." The next day she heard him tell a visitor that he was receiving an antacid to decrease the amount of acid in his stomach. But on the following day he was NPO for some blood chemistries and called the nurse for a pain medication. When she explained that the blood would be drawn in about five minutes and that then he could have his antacid, he replied, "But I want something to stop this stomach pain." Further exploration revealed that he did not relate the antacid to pain relief. Although he possessed two accurate pieces of information he was unable without further assistance to see the relationship between them.

Between the ages of two and seven years the child's cognitive processes involve centering on a single, striking feature to the exclusion of other important aspects of a situation. This is demonstrated by John, four and one-half years old, who had painful dressing changes involving the use of saline on cotton balls to cleanse the outer area. When the nurse tried to acquaint him with the equipment by handing him a cotton ball, he began to cry and pushed the cotton away. Apparently he had centered on the cotton balls as the cause of pain. When the cotton touched his hand he reacted as he had during the dressing change. It was impossible to tell whether he had been conditioned to feel pain on contact with the cotton ball, or simply anticipated pain when he saw one. In any event he appeared to have focused on the cotton balls as an important factor in the cause of pain.

Also between two and seven years of age the child's tendency toward artificialism, defined as regarding things as the product of human creation, affects the meanings he ascribes to pain. One seven-year-old boy told the nurse who had just given him an injection that she was "mean" for doing that. He seemed to believe that the infliction of pain was deliberate and hostile and that the nurse had control over whether or not it was done.

Artificialism, centering and other characteristics of the various cognitive levels in children are also seen in adults. Fear, anxiety, alterations in the level of consciousness and other factors may result in a lowering of cognitive ability in the adult.

Powerlessness. The concept of powerlessness has been defined as the individual's feeling that his behavior cannot determine the outcomes or reinforcements he seeks (Seeman and Evans). When a person is faced with a situation over which he believes he has little control he may cease to seek further information about his predicament. Why should he obtain knowledge about something he can do nothing about? Prior to becoming ill the patient may have a sense of powerlessness about all aspects of health and illness. Feelings of powerlessness may also be created by the illness situation and reinforced by health personnel who tell the patient that they will do everything necessary for him and that he is to receive this passively. They give him little information about the cause of his illness or pain and what, if anything, he can do to help himself. This may well be one of the reasons a patient does not complain of pain since he may feel that the necessity for pain relief is determined and controlled by others. On the other hand, it could be the reason a patient complains frequently about his pain since he has not been told of various pain-relief measures such as positioning or distraction that he could utilize himself.

A prenatal class illustrates how health team members can create in the patient a sense of powerlessness. A physician in residency in obstetrics and a nurse from the prenatal clinic conducted this class of 15 members. During the class the physician listed on the blackboard three types of regional anesthetics that would be available to the mother during labor. Toward the end of the class one expectant mother asked if she would have a choice of these anesthetics and a choice in whether or not she received one. The nurse replied that by the time she needed it she would not care which one she received and that the physician would decide. Further, no mention was ever made of anything the laboring patient could do for herself to alleviate discomfort such as keeping her bladder empty, relaxing between contractions, trying various positions and having her husband rub her lower back. At the conclusion of the class one patient commented, "This sounds terrible. I guess all I can do is go home and practice my Lamaze." Although she had found her own resource for pain relief, her comment contained an element of doubt about its usefulness, a doubt that may have been generated by this prenatal class. For the other patients without their own resources for pain relief, one wonders about the extent to which this class engendered fear and helplessness and what effect these feelings had on their labors.

Feelings of powerlessness, whether possessed by the patient initially or created by the situation, probably will result in the patient's knowing little about how to achieve pain relief, and may also foster fantasies about the cause and meaning of pain.

Presence, attitudes and feelings of others. When a patient is in pain or fears pain the simple presence of another person may influence his behavioral responses or his subjective experience. As mentioned previously a particular sociocultural group may have certain expectations regarding the people to whom the patient complains of pain. Consequently the patient may be more expressive about his pain in the presence of a nurse or physician than he is with family or friends, or the patient may be less expressive in the presence of anyone than when he is alone. For another patient the presence of someone may reduce loneliness and anxiety resulting from pain. In the United States the patient who tends to be very expressive because of the expectations of his culture may be influenced to behave in a more controlled manner because health team members with Old American attitudes convey to the patient that they find such expression of pain annoying.

The patient's behavioral responses to pain may also be influenced by the nurse's or physician's attitude concerning whether or not the patient should expect and experience pain. Such an expectation was conveyed by the leaders of the prenatal class described in the last section. Throughout the class both the physician and nurse consistently referred to uterine contractions as "pains." The physician described the frequency of these "pains" throughout labor, and ended by saying that when labor was progressing well the "pains" would be two to three minutes apart. One expectant mother immediately asked how long this part would last. When the physician replied, "Five to eight hours," the audience gasped in unison. The mother certainly should be told to expect some notable discomfort during labor. However, the lack of additional information, the emphasis on "pain" from the very beginning of labor, and the frequent use of the word "pain" seemed to produce a greater fear of pain than was necessary. The fact that the nurse and physician were personable and obviously eager to help did little to allay this fear.

Feelings of fear and anxiety in those who come in contact with the patient can cause or increase the patient's own fear and anxiety. This is especially important because fear and anxiety usually increase the subjective experience of pain. Some degree of these feelings almost always accompanies pain. However, a high degree of anxiety or fear may cause the patient to perceive a greater sensation of pain, intensify his behavioral responses and make it even more difficult for him to utilize his usual methods of coping with pain. This occurs in both the adult and the child patient. The following discussion will focus on the child since it is easy to observe others communicate fear and anxiety to the child and since the effects on the child are rather remarkable.*

Nurses, doctors and parents appear to experience a discomfort of their own when a child is in pain, particularly if they have had some part in causing that pain. The adult senses that the child depends upon him for assistance and protection. When the adult cannot provide this to the child's satisfaction the adult sometimes feels helpless and inadequate. Since the child often cannot understand what is happening to him and cannot comprehend the therapeutic or diagnostic merit of a procedure or the reason for his illness, some of his responses may tend to increase the adult's feelings of failure. The child may strike out at the adult, blame the adult for his pain, scream for help or cry loudly.

When the adult is concerned about the child and wants to help him, this type of behavior in the child can be very disturbing. It is at this point that the adult, rather than continuing in a kind and caring manner, may become angry with his own feelings of failure and in turn become angry with the child. The adult may convey this to the child in many ways. For example, he may restrain the child more firmly than necessary, increasing the child's feelings of being punished and purposely harmed. The adult may tell him to stop crying, showing very little understanding and acceptance of the child's point of view. In a way the adult who tells the child to stop crying is merely attempting to erase the signs of his inability to help the child. This expression of anger toward the child seems to be even more intense when the adult involved is unsure of his own competence in performing the procedure or giving care.

This can be illustrated by a nurse who packed an infected wound on Susan, six years old. She approached Susan pleasantly and explained very simply what she was going to do. As she proceeded Susan began to cry quietly. Very kindly the nurse said, "I don't mean to hurt you. Now don't cry." Susan attempted to stop crying by biting her lips. In a few seconds the nurse became obviously embarrassed over having forgotten some necessary dressings and medication. Her anxiety was evident in her curt tone of voice when she asked another nurse to bring her the supplies. Susan immediately began to move her legs slightly and the nurse called an aide to hold the child's legs firmly. Then Susan began to cry loudly and another nurse was called to hold her hands and arms. In this example, the child's behavior became more intense and less controlled as the nurse's anger and anxiety increased.

---

*The following material on the child is either a direct quote or adapted from McCaffery, Margo. "Brief Episodes of Pain in Children," *Current Concepts in Clinical Nursing,* Vol. II, Eds. Betty S. Bergersen, *et al.* St. Louis: C. V. Mosby Co., pp. 181-182, 1969.

A parent who is highly anxious about his child's illness and has a strong need to prevent further harm to the child can sometimes increase the child's fear. In the child's presence the parent may question the necessity of a procedure or cry about it. The parent can make the impending procedure seem even more ominous and punitive to the child. On the other hand, when the parent is able to handle his own feelings, he can focus on helping his child.

Threat to life situation.   Most of the other factors that influence the pain sensation and response culminate to produce what many people feel is the most significant influence on the patient's pain experience— the meaning of the pain to the patient. Beecher's (1956; b) now classic and much-quoted study gives dramatic support to the notion that the perceived intensity of pain and the behavioral responses to pain are largely determined by what the pain means to the patient. He compared a group of men who had wartime casualties with a group of male civilian patients who had comparable wounds. The soldiers had extensive injuries, were mentally alert and were not in shock. When they were questioned only 32% of them said they had enough pain to want anything done about it. By contrast 85% of the civilian patients desired narcotics for their pain. This study found no significant relationship between the extent of injury and the pain experienced, nor were there differences between sudden injury and chronic illness. These results have been interpreted to mean that the soldier's pain was associated with an improvement in his life situation; that is, he was removed from combat and safely returned to a hospital. On the other hand, the civilian's pain was associated with an unfavorable change in his life situation and threatened his life style. To him, pain implied death or serious illness. But to the soldier pain meant escape from a greater threat and this decreased his complaints of pain and perhaps also the perceived intensity of pain. Therefore, when pain threatens the patient's life situation, it appears that the patient will tend to experience a greater intensity of pain, complain more about the pain, and react more intensely.

Pain as a personal threat.   The possible or actual threat that pain poses for the patient may take several forms. First, it may threaten the patient's very life. He may fear that the undiagnosed pain in his head is a brain tumor that will lead to his death. Or, he may know that the pain in his abdomen is from a malignancy that will cause his death in a few months. In other words, the pain may mean possible or certain death.

Second, the pain may not imply a fatal illness but may be indicative of an actual or possible serious illness that will threaten the patient's activities of daily living. Or, the patient may not associate his pain with a serious illness, but the pain itself may be severe enough to hamper daily living. Role performance, such as that of breadwinner or mother, may be threatened by severe pain or pain associated with serious illness. Pain may also interfere with interpersonal relationships. Sexual activity may be painful if the patient has a back injury. Or, the irritability caused by the pain may prevent him from socializing with others. In addition the pain or the treatment for the pain may preclude the enjoyment of other activities such as eating, hiking, bathing or pursuing some hobby. Very simply, pain may mean to the patient that he has lost or will lose some of the pleasures of daily living.

Third, pain may be associated with a threat to the patient's body image. Pain may remind the patient of the recent or impending loss of a leg, the uterus or an eye. The pain from accidental lacerations of the face or from extensive burns over the body may mean possible scarring and loss of beauty.

The threat of pain often involves the fear of a loss or the experience of a loss, and therefore may be associated with the affects of anxiety, fear, depression or grief. For example, the patient's fear may be related to the objective threat that the pain in his leg indicates loss of the leg by amputation. Anxiety may result when pain threatens to deprive the patient of something he regards as valuable and perhaps essential to his existence as a person, such as loss of the ability to be creative or to earn money. Depression and possibly suicide results when the patient feels that pain has caused important losses such as the ability to enjoy daily living, when his self-esteem is lowered, and when he feels helpless to do anything about it. Grief and mourning occur when he tries to relinquish the losses he has incurred by pain.

Mrs. Lane, a 25-year-old postpartum patient, demonstrates the anxiety that can be associated with the meaning of pain and how this affects the patient's pain experience. Two weeks after the birth of her baby Mrs. Lane called her physician and reported to the office nurse that she had severe, diffuse pain in the perineal area that included cramping and burning sensations when she voided. An appointment was made for that day. She arrived in a wheelchair used to transport her from the car to the office. The patient said the pain was so severe she could not walk. While the nurse was with her in the examining room waiting for the physician, Mrs. Lane asked, "What do you suppose this is? Do you think I'll need surgery? I don't know what I'm going to do about the baby." Her behavior indicated anxiety about the implications of the pain. She seemed to fear that she might have some serious illness that would threaten her mothering role and cause her to lose the pleasure of caring for her baby. The physician diagnosed her problem as cystitis, gave her prescriptions for medication, and explained that the sulfisoxazole would control the infection and the Pyridium would alleviate the pain in the meantime. Mrs. Lane told the nurse good-bye with a smile and started to walk out of the office. When the nurse asked if she would like her wheelchair, Mrs. Lane replied, "I don't think I need it. The doctor says I'll be all right now." Her anxiety seemed to have disappeared, and she either did not perceive the pain as intensely as before or did not need to react to it any more. This illustrates how the patient can bear pain more easily when hope is high, the end can be seen and the reason for the pain is clear (Farnsworth) and how pain responses are more intense when pain threatens the life situation.

Perceptual dominance of pain. When a patient is experiencing pain and another source of pain is imposed on him, one of the pain sensations may become dominant and alter the perceived intensity of the other pain sensation. When the patient experiences intense pain in one area of the body, the threshold of sensory perception in other areas is raised (Berlin, Goodell and Wolff). In other words, intense pain in one area of the body causes the patient to be less sensitive to a milder pain in another area of the body. In fact, he may not feel the milder sensation. The presence of pain may also raise the thresholds of perception for other sensory inputs such as hearing, vibration and temperature.

Mrs. Helms, for example, who experienced a severe migraine headache during her hospitalization for a broken arm, demonstrated increased thresholds for milder pain and for auditory stimulation. When the nurse entered the room to administer an injection of ergotamine, she asked Mrs. Helms to turn to her side. The nurse's tone of voice was the one she ordinarily used in conversing with Mrs. Helms. However, Mrs. Helms did not respond until the request was repeated in a louder voice. After the injection the nurse told Mrs. Helms that she could turn to her back again. Mrs. Helms asked, "But aren't you going to give me something?" When the nurse said she had already given the injection, Mrs. Helms said she did not feel it. The perceptual dominance of her headache made her less sensitive than usual to the milder pain sensation of the injection and to auditory input.

If one pain sensation is not sufficiently intense to gain dominance over another, the patient may be aware of both pain sensations at the level of intensity he would perceive if they occurred separately. In general, pain intensity is not increased by the summation of impulses from noxious stimulation at different sites (Hardy). Therefore, multiple minor injuries do not result in excruciating pain. For example, in a hypothetical situation a patient has five lacerations, each causing a pain intensity equal to an arbitrary value of two. The patient will tend to perceive pain at the value of two rather than ten. The intensities of the lacerations are not added together to cause overwhelming pain.

Basic algesic types. One of the perceptual responses that has been correlated with pain responses is magnitude estimation. If an individual makes errors in the estimation of size, for example, he tends to be consistent in the direction of his errors. Thus, one person will almost always overestimate size while another repeatedly underestimates size. Relationships have been found between the direction of error and the person's tolerance for pain and sensory isolation. On the basis of these findings three algesic types were identified: reducers, augmenters and moderates. Reducers tend to decrease subjectively what they perceive. Therefore reducers tolerate pain well because they underestimate the intensity of pain. On the other hand, they are intolerant of sensory isolation because they apparently diminish even further the minimal sensory input. It follows that augmenters, because they tend to overestimate input, do not tolerate pain well but tolerate sensory isolation. Moderates alter only slightly what they perceive and tend to be moderately tolerant of both pain and isolation (Petrie, Collins and Solomon).

While the inverse relationship between the ability to endure pain and the ability to tolerate sensory isolation has not been supported by others (Peters, *et al.*), the importance of these findings is that a person may have a consistent perceptual style. That is, an individual's judgments of external stimuli, including pain, may consistently err in one direction or the other. Although it would be difficult, if not impossible, to change permanently the patient's perceptual style, these findings suggest that any temporary measure such as drugs that causes the patient to reduce subjectively what he perceives will result in pain relief or increased tolerance for pain.

What are the relationships between or the combined effects of several influencing factors?

Once the nurse has assessed the factors that seem to influence the patient's pain sensation and response, it is pertinent to later plans for intervention to identify two characteristics of the influencing factors. One may be that several of the influencing factors have a common theme. For example, the nurse may have ascertained that the patient is subjected to sensory restriction in the form of perceptual monotony that tends to increase his sensitivity to pain; that as a result of the traditions of his culture and his own past experience with pain the patient has developed a method of handling pain that involves the use of other people as a means of distracting him from pain; and that the feelings and presence of his friend, who is the only visitor, inhibit socializing because the friend conveys his anxiety about the patient's condition by insisting that the patient rest and not talk while he is there. The common theme in these influencing factors is the patient's need for social stimulation. When a common theme such as this has been identified, intervention can be focused on this element. Intervention will be more efficient, more specific to the patient's needs and hopefully more effective.

A second characteristic of two or more influencing factors is their combined effect. In other words, they may tend to reinforce each other and have more than a simple additive effect upon the patient's pain experience. For example, the nurse's assessment may reveal that the patient has feelings of powerlessness because he has not been engaged in making decisions about his care, including pain relief measures. In addition, he has not been given any information about pain-relief measures or how he could participate in his care. These two influencing factors reinforce each other. Feelings of powerlessness often cause the patient to fail to obtain information, in turn perpetuating the failure of others to give him information, and further reinforcing his feelings of powerlessness.

In another situation the patient fears that his pain is indicative of a fatal illness, and at the same time others convey to him their anxiety about the significance of his pain. The patient will experience a far greater amount of anxiety about pain than he would if only one of these factors were present. The conditions reinforce each other to produce a mushrooming effect, not just an additive effect. When the nurse recognizes such a situation, her intervention can be focused on the immediate control of one of the factors.

Further Exploration

Physiological factors. With regard to the specificity theory of pain, the notion that the undifferentiated free nerve endings are pain-specific receptors has largely been abandoned since at least some of these receptors may also subserve warmth, cold and touch (Sternbach, 1968). Loewenstein, however, provides some evidence in favor of receptor specificity. The issue of pain-specific fibers is similar to that of receptors. The A-delta and C fibers also transmit touch and temperature impulses, and apparently fibers other than these may transmit pain (Sternbach, 1968).

Some opponents of the gate control theory state that it is an unsubstantiated concept and that the notion of cells in the substantia gelatinosa that inhibit transmission is purely speculative. Others say that the theory ignores spinal root modulation by antidromic blocking ("Pain," 1970). The reader may wish to pursue the debate of this theory by examining the proceedings of the Harvey Cushing Society meeting in 1971.

The nature of the noxious stimulation capable of eliciting pain has been the subject of some theorizing. Hardy suggests that pain results when noxious stimulation begins to damage the pain-fiber ending and that pain is an indication of the rate of tissue damage. Therefore, extensive wounds may be painless if no further tissue damage is occurring, and slight wounds may be extremely painful if there is a progressive increase in tissue damage. Accordingly, high-intensity pain can be maintained only for a short period of time since it reflects rapid death of tissue and pain endings. Therefore, high intensity intractable pain over a long period of time is felt to be an impossibility. Such pain is explained as ordinarily nonpainful sensations that the individual under stress interprets as painful and unacceptable.

Some researchers have attempted to identify the chemical agents that produce pain. The swelling and vasodilation accompanying inflammation that follows injury seems insufficient to cause all of the pain. Tissue and serum breakdown products could be the cause of pain. The accumulation of red and white corpuscles along with other agents provide conditions favorable to the formation of bradykinin or bradykinin-like peptides. Bradykinin evokes pain when it stimulates receptors (Lim). Others have postulated pain-producing substance (PPS) that is somewhat like bradykinin (Armstrong,*et al*).

Cultural factors. Blaylock summarizes several studies on the perception and reaction thresholds of various groups such as the Negroes, Italians, Russians, Jews, American Indians, Eskimos, prize fighters and coal miners. The results of these studies may be helpful in understanding patients' behavioral responses and in devising appropriate controls for nursing research on pain. Additional studies by Sternbach and Tursky (1965; Tursky and Sternbach, 1967) indicate that culturally acquired attitudes are paralleled by physiological activity in the form of heart rate, skin resistance and diphasic palmar skin potentials. For example, when groups of Yankee, Irish, Jewish and Italian housewives were compared, the Yankee women showed a significantly more rapid and greater decrease in the number of diphasic palmar skin potentials.

Psychological factors. With regard to the effects on pain of emotionally traumatic life experiences and secondary gains, it is interesting to note Wolff's (1953) observations on headaches. He estimates that about 90% of the vascular and muscle tension headaches severe enough to be brought to the attention of a physician are manifestations of life stress, anger and striving. He suggests that headaches and some other painful symptoms are inappropriate patterns of reaction to social pressures. But these patterns may be followed indefinitely in spite of the fact that they do not bring fulfillment.

The fact that emotionally traumatic life experiences and secondary gains of pain may establish the painful symptoms as exceptionally useful to the individual may be related to the success or failure of various pain relief measures. Recent clinical results of the use of electroanalgesia on patients with intractable pain suggest that the patient's personality is a determining variable in the effectiveness of this procedure ("Pain," 1970).

The studies cited in this chapter suggest that, in general, past experiences with pain result in the patient's being more sensitive to and more threatened by pain. Further evidence for this is a study by Melzack and Scott, not included previously in this chapter because the conditions of this study are not likely to occur in human beings. Groups of dogs raised in isolation were compared to dogs raised in a rather normal environment. At maturity the dogs were subjected to various noxious stimuli and it was found that the restricted dogs showed reflex responses to pain but did not know how to make the proper avoidance responses. In fact, many of the restricted dogs remained closer to the experimenter after the noxious stimuli were used then they had before they were applied. The authors concluded that the meaning of pain and attitudes toward pain are a function of early experiences with pain. Indeed avoidance pain responses appear to *require* a background of early and prolonged experiences with pain.

An understanding of the various stages of cognitive development in the child is very useful in the nursing care of children with pain. It is also helpful in the care of adults with pain since many factors may lower the adult's cognitive ability. Piaget, a developmental psychologist, is credited with having done the most extensive work in the area of the stages of intellectual development in children. A summary of his work, begun some 30 years ago, is available in a book by Flavell. A briefer summary with a focus on application to nursing intervention has been prepared by this author (McCaffery, 1968).

Since the concept of powerlessness is also applicable to many areas of nursing care besides pain, the reader may wish to pursue this in Johnson's article. She discusses some of the research, problems in assessment of powerlessness, application of the concept to nursing care and other aspects of the topic.

Sternbach's (1968) review of the literature suggests that perceptual factors other than magnitude estimation may be related to behavioral responses to pain. Based on a subject's performance on a rod alignment task he may be judged field-dependent or field-independent. The field-independent person uses internal cues to make judgments and the field-dependent uses external cues. The field-independent person demonstrates high pain reactivity and both sympathetic and parasympathetic responses. The field-dependent person shows low pain reactivity and primarily parasympathetic responses.

Anxiety has been mentioned and implied throughout this chapter, and most of the time it has been treated as an independent variable. In other words, the focus has been the effect of anxiety on pain responses, not the effect of pain on anxiety. For the most part, the type of anxiety discussed has been situational anxiety rather than trait anxiety. Trait anxiety, which can be measured in several ways such as the Taylor Manifest Anxiety Scale, is a personality factor that is a relatively enduring characteristic of the person. Trait anxiety as well as situational anxiety may be important variables to control in nursing research on pain. In any event, the differences between the pain responses of subjects with and without trait anxiety reaffirm the importance of differentiating between tolerance for pain and evaluation of pain intensity. In some studies introverts were considered to have the trait of anxiety and extroverts were not. It was found that introverts had a lesser tolerance for pain but that extroverts gave more exaggerated descriptions of pain. Trait anxiety has also been correlated with persistent pains (Sternbach, 1968).

Chapter 4

Nursing Diagnosis of the Patient with Pain

Chapters 2 and 3 discuss the nurse's assessment of the patient's behavioral responses to pain and her assessment of the factors that influence the patient's sensation of pain and response to pain. This assessment of the patient constitutes the *process* of nursing diagnosis. The *statement* of the nursing diagnosis is discussed in this chapter.

The particular statement of the nursing diagnosis proposed in this chapter is one the author has found useful in the nursing care of patients with pain. It summarizes the assessment of the patient, and it points the way to nursing intervention since it specifies many of the factors influencing the patient's pain experience. Sometimes more than one statement of the nursing diagnosis is necessary if the patient experiences more than one type of pain. For example, when the patient has several different pains such as headache associated with the side effects of a drug, chest pain due to empyema and pain in the inguinal area due to an abscess, a separate nursing diagnosis usually is made for each pain.

What are the parts of the nursing diagnosis?

In brief, the nursing diagnosis statement contains four interrelated parts: (1) the type of pain, (2) the factors that influence the existence and characteristics of the pain sensation, (3) the patient's behavioral responses to the pain experience and (4) the factors that influence the patient's behavioral responses. The first two parts of the diagnosis comprise a unit analyzing the patient's pain sensation. The last two parts are another unit analyzing the patient's behavior. These two units will be discussed separately.

But before discussing each unit of the diagnosis, it is perhaps pertinent to acknowledge that this type of nursing diagnosis is rather cumbersome. It is certainly more lengthy than the physician's usual diagnostic statement. However, medicine is much older as a profession than is nursing. Nursing is beginning to identify many areas of patient problems. But in general the appropriate terminology has not yet been developed to convey in one or two words the symptoms, cause and probable type of intervention related to a patient's problem. When the physician diagnoses detached retina, for example, we know at once (or can find a reference that tells us) the general signs and symptoms, probable causes, possible types of treatment and even the prognosis. On the other hand, when the nurse is caring for a patient with a problem such as pain, no combination of any two or three words will tell physicians or other nurses the cause of the pain, the type of pain, the patient's responses to pain and the reasons for these responses, not to mention possible intervention and the prognosis for pain relief or tolerance. Therefore, the nurse is left with an unwieldy statement of the nursing diagnosis that is, at best, several sentences long.

The painful sensation and the factors that influence its existence and characteristics. These are the two parts that comprise the first unit of the nursing diagnosis. Assuming that the nurse's assessment has been comprehensive, she already knows the characteristics of the patient's painful sensation and which factors influence the existence and characteristics of the pain. Now she must organize this information into one or several sentences.

The type of painful sensation is described in terms of its intensity, quality, location, duration and intermittency. Two examples of statements of this portion of the nursing diagnosis are:

1. Mr. Sanders has moderately severe, aching pain in the right upper abdominal area of ten days' duration, increasing in severity when he performs certain physical activities.

2. Bobby has mild pricking and moderate to severe aching pain in the left and right gluteal muscle areas four to five times a day occurring over the last seven days. The mild pricking pain lasts about two seconds, the severe aching pain about two to five minutes, and the moderate aching pain about two minutes.

The next portion of this unit of the nursing diagnosis concerns the factors that influence the existence of the pain and the characteristics of it. This identifies the cause of a painful sensation and what alters or causes the characteristics of the pain. Continuing with the two examples above, this portion may be stated as follows:

1. Mr. Sanders' pain has an aching quality because it is visceral. The pain sensation is located in the right upper abdominal area in the region of the liver. It is associated with cellular damage and swelling in the liver due to the presence of filterable virus B. An increase in intensity of pain is caused by physical strain in the form of pressure on the liver

from contraction of surrounding skeletal muscles and pressure from nearby viscera. This increased intensity of pain is evoked when the patient engages in certain activities such as sitting up from the supine position. The general level of intensity at which he perceives pain may be· increased because of the threat of pain to his life situation. He comments that he is unable to enjoy many of the pleasures of daily living and his environment is usually perceptually monotonous. Theoretically the pain mechanism could be explained in terms of the slowly conducting fiber system that carries the pain impulses being dominant over the rapidly conducting fiber system that inhibits the transmission of pain impulses.

2. Bobby's pain is located in the gluteal muscle area because this is where injections are given that cause swelling in the muscle and pressure on surrounding tissues. The pricking quality is a result of piercing the skin with a needle. The intensity is mild because a small needle is used. The aching quality is associated with the swelling and pressure in deeper tissues. It is of moderate intensity because a relatively large amount of 2 cc's is injected each time. The intensity is severe when the 2 cc's is injected in an inflamed area where other injections have been given, increasing the amount of swelling and pressure. An increase in the perceived intensity of pain may occur and be related to the fact that Bobby has a cognitive ability typical of his age of three years. This prevents him from possessing an understanding of the purpose of the injections. Four of the daily injections are antibiotics, but a fifth injection of a sedative is given on some days. The sedative is in preparation for chest x-rays because he reacts with extreme fear to the x-ray procedure. He may fear that each injection will be followed by an x-ray. This may heighten his anxiety about each injection and thereby increase the perceived intensity of pain. Theoretically the pain mechanism may be explained as an open gate to transmission of pain signals because of lack of stimulation to the inhibitory cutaneous afferents and because descending fibers from the brain interpret the sensation as pain on the basis of past experiences with pain and the possible meaning of the pain.

These last two patient examples are rather lengthy because an attempt has been made to be thorough in identifying factors that influence the existence and characteristics of the pain sensation. This degree of thoroughness is helpful to the nurse who is beginning to learn how to apply her knowledge about pain and organize the information she obtained in her assessment of the individual patient. However, such thoroughness is not always of practical value in actual nursing care. For example, in the case of Bobby, the nurse may know very well what causes the existence and characteristics of pain associated with injections, and she may choose to eliminate an explanation of this in the statement of the nursing diagnosis. On the other hand, in the case of Mr. Sanders, the nurse may not have understood some of the reasons for the existence and characteristics of pain associated with serum hepatitis. It may be a valuable aid to her and other nurses to include this in her statement of the nursing diagnosis. The nurse may also wish to eliminate a theoretical explanation of the pain mechanism when she feels she comprehends this aspect. But her understanding of possible pain mechanisms will be valuable when she plans nursing intervention.

The patient's behavioral responses to the pain experience and the factors that influence his behavioral responses. These are the two parts of the second unit of the nursing diagnosis. Again, the nurse's assessment has provided her with this information. Her task now is to organize it into one or several sentences. The patient's behavioral responses are stated for each phase of the pain experience; that is, the anticipation of pain, the actual pain sensation and the aftermath of pain. However, there are no noticeable anticipation and aftermath phases if the patient has a continuous and stable intensity of pain. In another patient there may be anticipation and aftermath phases that are not free of pain but surround an increased intensity of pain. Mr. Sanders, for example, seems to have pain constantly but he anticipates an increased intensity of pain when he engages in certain physical activities.

The patient's behavioral responses to the pain experience may be numerous. Therefore, it is more practical to include in the statement of the nursing diagnosis only those that are most easily observed and/or the most frequently occurring. Sometimes a behavioral response that does not fit either or both of these criteria is pertinent to include because it is indicative of what the patient is experiencing. For example, it may be rare to observe a particular patient crying about pain, but he may confess one time to another nurse that he cries when he is alone. Or, another patient may say only once that every time he experiences severe pain he is afraid he has a terrible disease. Neither of these examples is easy to observe or occurs frequently, but both are pertinent and should be included in the statement of the nursing diagnosis.

Following are examples of statements for the behavioral responses to pain made by the two patients, Mr. Sanders and Bobby, previously discussed in this chapter:

1. Upon questioning Mr. Sanders rates his constant pain as "some" (rated on a scale of none, a little bit, some, quite a bit or a lot). He frequently and voluntarily describes it as feeling "like someone is hitting me in the stomach." Pain associated with movement is "quite a bit." Behavior accompanying his constant pain consists of failure to initiate conversation, little attention to the environment and a blank

stare. When he anticipates pain from movement or pressure he wrinkles his forehead and moves his hand to shield the upper right abdominal area of pain. This facial expression continues during the period of increased pain intensity and his face appears pale. Following this increased intensity of pain he remains quite still, sometimes closes his eyes for a few seconds and he may not respond when spoken to. His overall pattern of handling pain appears to consist of these minimally expressive responses.

2. Bobby's anticipation of pain begins whenever he sees a nurse enter the room with a tray of medications. He begins to whimper quietly and pulls the covers up around him. When the nurse touches him to position him he cries loudly, screams "no," and pulls away from her. This behavior continues through the period of the injection except that he cries even louder while the medication is being injected. After the injection is over he whimpers quietly, pulls the covers up around him and watches the doorway. If he is left alone, this continues for up to five minutes. His overall pattern of handling pain seems to be a combination of vocalizations and escape movements, or flight responses.

The last part of the statement of the nursing diagnosis concerns why the patient behaves as he does. There are many other ways in which each of the above patients could behave. Bobby might try to hit the nurse or he might remain very quiet throughout the injection and bite his lip to keep from crying. Mr. Sanders might frequently moan and cry with his pain or angrily tell the nurse that she is hurting him when she assists him in sitting up. Therefore, the nurse wants to identify the factors that influence the patient to respond to pain in his own particular manner. For the sake of brevity and practicality the statement of the nursing diagnosis usually contains those factors that are major determinants of the patient's behavior and especially those that are pertinent to nursing management of pain. For the purpose of providing adequate illustrations of statements of this part of the diagnosis, the following examples for Mr. Sanders and Bobby are more lengthy and inclusive than is usually necessary:

1. Mr. Sanders, age 40, behaves in accordance with many of the expectations of the Old American cultural group. Therefore, he is generally nonexpressive about his pain and able to describe the sensation objectively. The fact that he experiences visceral rather than cutaneous pain adds to the tendency to remain quiet. The long duration of his pain (ten days) and fatigue from both pain and sleep interruptions increase his tendency to pay little attention to the environment. The high intensity of pain on movement may account for his increased threshold for auditory stimulation. The sharp but short intensity of pain on movement causes pallor since blood is shifting from superficial vessels to other organs. When he anticipates pressure or certain

physical activities, he wrinkles his forehead, attempts to shield the area of pain and becomes physically inactive afterwards. He responds in this way because past experience has taught him when to anticipate pain and that additional movement or external pressure will prolong or increase the intensity of pain.

2. In Bobby's past experiences with pain his relatively low level of cognitive ability has caused him to focus on only a few striking features of the event. The sight of the nurse with a medication tray causes him to anticipate pain even when he does not receive an injection. He is anxious about the threat of the injection because he has focused on the injection as being a cue for going to x-ray. Anxiety is also increased by his mother's anxiety over injections when she is present. This high level of anxiety plus his mother's acceptance of his behavior leads to the highly expressive vocalizations about the pain experience. The fact that the pain is initially cutaneous and is imposed externally accounts for his flight reactions of pulling away from the nurse and pulling the covers up around him. The moderate to severe intensity of the pain of injecting the medication results in increased loudness of crying.

Since examples have been given separately for each of the four parts of the nursing diagnosis, some facts have been stated more than once. When the four parts are combined, this redundancy can be eliminated and the statement of the nursing diagnosis will be briefer.

How is the statement of the nursing diagnosis used in the nursing care plan?

The nursing diagnosis, stated according to the previous suggestions, identifies and describes the patient's need or problem. For this reason the nursing diagnosis is usually one part of the nursing care plan. Even if the diagnosis is not formally labeled as part of the nursing care plan, it is nevertheless basic to the formulation of a plan of intervention for the particular patient.

It is necessary for the nurse to communicate to other health team members her nursing diagnosis of the patient. In doing this she adds to the amount of information others possess about the patient. Others may consider this information along with their own assessments of the patient. Sharing information will enable each nurse caring for the patient to formulate more effective nursing intervention.

The nurse's assessment and diagnosis of the patient with pain may have been done mentally or in writing, but how she communicates this for the purpose of improving patient care will vary in different situations. Some nurses may work in agencies that provide forms on which all of the assessment as well as the statement of the nursing diagnosis may be written. But the reality of the situation is that many nurses work in agencies that provide a two by four-inch space, if that much, for what may be called "nursing measures."

Whether or not the nursing diagnosis for the patient with pain is included in the nursing care plan and how the diagnosis is communicated is not only a matter of writing space. It is also determined by the philosophy of nursing care actually practiced by the agency and by the attitudes of other nurses and health team members within the agency. The health care agency's philosophy may be that the best nursing care consists only of thorough physical care and performance of activities delegated by the physicians. If this is the priority and if no more nurses are employed than are required to do this, a written nursing diagnosis about the patient in pain is not likely to have much influence on the behavior of any nurse except the one who wrote it. Or, if nurses and health team members are accustomed to oral communication of the more individualized aspects of nursing care, a written nursing diagnosis may be largely unnoticed. It may be regarded as time-consuming, unnecessary and somewhat disrespectful of the rapport that has been established between the health team members. In another instance health team members may acquire most of their information through observation of what others do, and a nursing diagnosis may be best communicated to them by the nurse's daily nursing care practices.

While the author favors the use of a written nursing diagnosis that can be shared by all health team members, it is the care the patient receives and the effect this has on him that is most important. When the nurse wants to share with other health team members what she knows about the patient and his pain, she must communicate it in a way that will result in the greatest improvement in the patient's ability to handle his pain.

The nurse may find that a statement of her nursing diagnosis has more meaning to health team members if she directly relates her diagnosis to nursing intervention. Various parts of the nursing diagnosis may be used to support the rationale for the intervention. In the author's experience, this type of nursing care plan is more acceptable and understandable to most health team members. It focuses on specific types of intervention for the patient and briefly gives the reasons why the intervention seems to be indicated for the particular patient.

Further Exploration

Much has been said about whether or not nursing care plans are valuable. In any situation where it is possible, this author favors the use of written nursing care plans for every patient. However, this opinion is not shared by all nurses. Harris suggests that nursing care plans are more important for certain types of patients than others. Among those who need nursing care plans are patients who are deaf or who will not ask for help. On the other hand, she refutes those reasons so often given for not writing a nursing care plan. For example, the nurse who says she does not have the time to write a care plan may not know how to write it or may not feel that it is as important as the other things she must do. And the nurse who says the information is communicated orally may be in error when there is much turnover in the nursing staff or when patients are frequently transferred from one area of the hospital to another.

Palisin says that "nursing care plans are a snare and a delusion." She discusses several reasons why nursing care plans are not written, maintained or used. She believes that the written nursing care plan is a burden to the practitioner and that it often hinders individualized nursing care.

Chapter | 5

Nursing Intervention During the Three Phases of Pain: Anticipation, Presence, Aftermath

The assumptions underlying efforts to relieve a patient's pain are based upon ethical and humanitarian as well as strictly medical considerations. From an objective, medical viewpoint pain relief is advisable because responses to pain may have harmful physiological effects such as strain on certain organs that may impede recovery from illness and may even be fatal. Postoperative pain may cause shock. If pain prevents the patient from cooperating with coughing, ambulation and other activities, pulmonary complications may occur.

Finally, pain relief is important in that it allows the patient to fulfill his total potential. In drawing attention to itself pain prevents involvement in other life experiences. Therefore, pain relief is desirable because it allows the patient to live a full life.

How is nursing intervention logically derived?

Individualized nursing intervention for the patient in pain is naturally determined by the nursing assessment. One part of it is designed to manage as many as possible of the factors that influence the patient's behavior and pain sensation. That is, to alter factors that cause or increase the pain sensation, and to alter those factors that cause or increase the intensity of the patient's behavioral responses to pain. For example, if physical strain on the incision increases pain, nursing intervention may be designed to lessen or eliminate that physical strain. If the patient's behavioral response to this pain is intensified because he knows someone whose incision "broke open" and if he fears this will happen to him, nursing intervention may be designed to lessen this fear with appropriate information. Other nursing activities, listed and discussed in this chapter, may also be employed to manage the factors that account for this patient's increased intensity of pain and his fear of the pain.

Another part of nursing intervention is based on the nursing assessment of the patient's behavioral responses to pain and the factors that influence his response style. It may not be possible, either immediately or eventually, to determine nursing intervention to manage the causes of the pain and the patient's response to it. The nurse must then design intervention that is an appropriate response to the patient's behaviors. For example, if pain is unavoidable and the patient cries, the nurse must determine whether to leave him alone to cry, ignore the crying but remain with him, or encourage him to cry. Her choice of these responses should be based on her understanding of the effectiveness of the crying as a coping mechanism and on her knowledge of the responses the patient has been conditioned to make as a result of cultural expectations and his own experiences.

What are the objectives of nursing intervention?

Pain relief is one of the overall goals of nursing intervention, but it is important to state the goal in less general terms. To begin with, for a particular patient, accomplishment of the goal may take any one of several forms: total elimination of pain; decrease in the intensity, duration and/or frequency of pain; increase in tolerance for pain; decrease in the anxiety associated with the anticipation and aftermath of pain; increase in general comfort; or recognition of and help for the patient who *needs* a certain degree of pain. These forms of the goal range from the patient for whom it is possible to eliminate pain entirely to the patient who does not desire pain relief. Between these two extremes are patients for whom the nurse can provide varying degrees of pain relief or general comfort. The assessment process will probably indicate which of these goals she may expect to achieve with the patient. In many cases total abolition of pain is impossible. A more realistic goal may be reduction of pain to a tolerable level or a lowering of anxiety preceding and following pain.

The objectives of nursing intervention are of a different order from the more generally stated goals. Objectives are stated in terms of behavioral outcomes. In this instance objectives may include the nurse's behavior (nurse-centered objectives) and the patient's behavior (patient-centered objectives). Specific and objective descriptions of the behavior expected of the nurse and the patient facilitate accomplishment of the behavioral outcome and evaluation of whether or not the objective has been achieved.

Nurse-centered objectives. Statements concerning the nurse's actions toward or in behalf of the patient are the most common objectives found in nursing care plans. They often take the form of suggestions such as how to position the patient most comfortably, when to administer an analgesic, or what to tell the patient about his pain. Basically, these are nurse-centered objectives because they describe what the nurse does. The nursing activities to be discussed in this chapter are also a form of nurse-centered objectives.

It is important for the nurse to determine precisely what she may do to assist a particular patient with pain. Although the nurse may state that the patient needs "emotional support" or "comfort measures," this cannot be accomplished unless the nurse can give a description of the nursing activities that meet these needs. Formulation of nurse-centered objectives, whether or not these objectives are written in a nursing care plan, is essential to the performance of any nursing care. Inability to describe nursing intervention is probably one reason nurses tend to do so little for the patient with pain. Both research and informal observation repeatedly confirm the idea that most nursing intervention related to pain is confined to the administration of an analgesic. This occurs in spite of the fact that most physicians expect more than this from the nurse. One way the nurse can improve the quality of care received by the patient with pain is to develop the ability to give objective descriptions of nursing activities. In this way she is more aware of exactly what she is doing. If the nursing care is effective, it can then be repeated. If the activity is not effective, the nurse may revise her objective and attempt another approach. Objective descriptions of effective nursing activities are also important because the nurse is able to communicate the care to others. If the nurse can describe exactly what she has done to provide pain relief for the patient, then other nurses will be able to do the same thing.

The performance of the nurse-centered objective is not an end in itself; it is only a means. The crux of nursing intervention is the patient-centered objective—what does the nurse expect to accomplish by acting in a particular way?

Patient-centered objectives. When the nurse performs an activity that is aimed at pain relief, she expects or hopes that the patient will show some evidence that his pain is indeed relieved. This evidence will be in the form of the patient's behavioral response such as a decrease in heart rate or his verbal confirmation that the pain is less severe. A statement that objectively describes the patient behavior indicating pain relief is a patient-centered objective. This particular patient response is the reason for formulating and performing the nurse-centered objective. It is the final test of the effectiveness of nursing care. As Smith suggests, the patient-centered objective tells the nurse where she is going and enables her to determine whether or not she got there.

A significant problem arises in formulating any patient-centered objectives, particularly those associated with evidence of pain relief. This problem is that the hoped-for or expected behavioral response from the patient must be based on the nurse's understanding of the factors that influence the particular patient's pattern of response to pain. Just as patients express pain differently, so will they express pain relief differently. And this may vary somewhat in the same patient from time to time. For example, following a pain relief measure one patient may sleep for two hours. At another time this same patient may begin to initiate conversation with his roommate and others who visit him. If this patient had cried quietly following a pain relief measure, it might mean that the pain was the same or even worse. On the other hand, if another patient had cried softly after lying rigidly in bed, it might indicate pain relief.

The point is that the nurse must be very careful in predicting what patient behavior will indicate pain relief in the individual patient at a particular time. The nurse must know the patient's usual responses to pain and pain relief and the reasons for these types of responses. The nurse also must not let her personal values and cultural orientation influence her expectations of patient behavior. For example, she may feel that the patient's loud screaming in response to pain is understandable in view of the intensity of the pain. Once the pain becomes considerably less intense, she may not easily accept the patient's moaning. But, depending upon this patient's past experiences and cultural conditioning, the nurse may be in error to expect a cessation of moaning unless the pain can be completely eliminated.

In spite of the problems with the nurse's own cultural orientation and the wide range of possible behavioral responses between patients and within the same patient, statements of patient-centered objectives are not impossible. Once these problems are recognized and the nurse has some experience with a particular patient, patient-centered objectives can be fairly accurate and realistic. At first the nurse may have to list several possible behavioral outcomes that could indicate pain relief in a given patient. Later she will be able to predict them more closely.

Some examples of patient-centered objectives follow. Note that patient behavior is objectively described, the approximate time of its occurrence is stated, and its duration is indicated. In a written nursing care plan, the nurse-centered objective precedes the patient-centered objective. In some of the following examples the nurse-centered objective is mentioned briefly.

1. About 5 minutes after Mr. Jones begins to play chess with his roommate, he will stop clenching his teeth and will not request an analgesic until the game is over.

2. Between 10 and 30 minutes after receiving an analgesic and being

held for the reading of a story, John will fall asleep for two hours.

3. Almost immediately after assuming a horizontal position, Mrs. Carter will, upon questioning, state that her headache is of moderate intensity rather than severe. This intensity will be maintained as long as she is lying down.

4. The next time Barbara has a spinal tap she will be placed on her back as soon as the procedure is over. Because she knows that there will be no further pain, she will stop crying when she is placed on her back.

5. While the nurse remains with Mrs. Powell and discusses her medical progress during the half hour prior to her daily wound debridement, Mrs. Powell's heart rate will be slower by eight to ten beats per minute and she will not perspire.

The first three patient-centered objectives deal with the period of the presence of pain. The last two objectives relate to the phases of aftermath and anticipation, respectively. When the patient experiences all three phases of pain, objectives are formulated for each phase.

What are some nursing activities that can be used to manage influencing factors and to serve as appropriate responses to patient behavior during the anticipation and/or presence of pain?

In this section the discussion of nursing management of the patient with pain is approached in terms of what the nurse actually does with and for the patient. These nursing activities are:

- establishing a relationship with the patient with pain
- teaching the patient about pain
- using the patient group situation
- managing other people who come in contact with the patient
- providing other sensory input
- promoting rest and relaxation
- using behavior therapy
- administering pharmacological agents
- administering placebos
- using waking-imagined analgesia
- decreasing noxious stimuli
- utilizing other professional assistance
- being with the patient.

These nursing activities are not mutually exclusive. For example, teaching the patient about pain may involve using patient groups or interacting with family members and others who come in contact with the patient. Also, as another example, any pain relief maneuver has a potential placebo effect. Therefore, these nursing activities overlap to a certain extent.

Principles of pain relief. The nursing activities are based upon various principles of providing pain relief. The major principles are: modifying anxiety associated with the pain experience, altering the amount or pattern of stimuli through major sensory modalities, eliciting behaviors that are incompatible with pain responses, and using what the patient believes will result in pain relief. Discussion and documentation of these and other closely related principles will be done in conjunction with certain nursing activities.

Some of the principles of nursing intervention will be referred to in relation to more than one nursing activity. For instance, the principle of eliciting behaviors that are incompatible with pain responses will be implicit or explicit in the discussion of activities such as assisting the patient to relax, to use waking-imagined analgesia, or to use distraction. And more than one principle may apply to a particular nursing activity. For example, the principles of incompatible behavior and of increasing sensory input both apply to distraction. This also demonstrates that many of the principles are intimately related, since increasing sensory input may elicit behaviors incompatible with pain.

Anxiety as a factor in pain experience. One of the most basic principles underlying the nursing management of the patient with pain is the modification of anxiety associated with the pain experience. Most other principles are related to this one to some extent. Therefore, it is important to clarify at the outset the general way in which pain relief is related to the interplay between anxiety and pain. *During the anticipation of pain, pain relief is enhanced if the patient experiences a moderate amount of anxiety and this anxiety is channeled into methods of coping with pain. When a pain sensation is felt, the reduction of anxiety associated with pain tends to decrease the perceived intensity of the sensation and/or increase the tolerance for pain.* These statements include two important phrases that must be understood. First, the reader will note that we are speaking of anxiety associated with pain, not anxiety about some unrelated event. In some cases anxiety about an event unrelated to pain may become related to pain. This may occur when the individual attempts to solve an unrelated problem by expressing his anxiety through his painful experience. Instances of this may be hypochondriacal pain or phantom pain. When anxiety becomes associated with pain, a reduction in this anxiety will contribute to pain relief. But, if anxiety remains associated with an event unrelated to pain, the unrelated event may act as a form of distraction when pain is present. This will decrease the perceived intensity of pain. For example, during the California earthquake of February, 1971, anxiety about the earthquake and after-shocks acted as a distractor from pain for some patients.

The second aspect of the previous statements that calls for elaboration is the difference in the desired level of anxiety during the anticipation and presence of pain. When pain is *felt*, anxiety associated with pain probably should be reduced to an absolute minimum. But the reduction of anxiety to this level during the *anticipation* of pain is not recommended. In fact, adequate preparation for impending pain practically precludes this possibility. The evidence suggests that a moderate level of anxiety is desirable during the period of anticipation of pain (Janis). Simply stated, the patient with moderate anxiety worries about his impending pain some of the time but not all of the time. This degree of worry, or moderate anxiety, seems to be necessary for the patient to be able to handle his pain. To promote pain relief we will assume that this moderate level of anxiety should be derived mostly from the patient's knowledge of what may actually occur. It should be derived minimally from the threat of the unknown or a threat to the essence of his personality.

The use of all the suggested nursing activities with all patients is not being advocated. Rather, the nurse must select for each patient those activities that will most effectively manage his behavioral responses and the factors that influence the pain sensation and response. The author recommends the use of a variety of nursing activities for pain relief besides the use of analgesics. The nursing activities accompanying the administration of an analgesic may be as important as or even more important than the medication itself. Also, sometimes an analgesic is contraindicated or does not provide sufficient pain relief. Therefore, the use of several appropriately selected nursing activities should provide greater and more dependable pain relief for the patient than he would receive if only one pain relief measure were employed.

Some authorities on various aspects of the subject of pain have interesting and convincing statements to make about the value of using a variety of pain relief measures. Keats found that postoperative patients request analgesics for many discomforts that could be relieved without an analgesic. These include backache, headache, uncomfortable position, sore throat and distended bladder. Similarly, Bochnak, Rhymes and Leonard found that many pain complaints could be relieved without the use of drugs. Further, they found that exploration of what the patient meant by his pain complaint increased the effectiveness of the analgesic. In accordance with this, Wolff and Wolf state that it is more important to deal with the patient's reaction to pain than with his perception of the pain.

In obstetrics, Chertok found that the use of the Lamaze method or other psychological methods of analgesia during labor and delivery produced several medical advantages. These advantages included a reduction in the length of labor and a lower incidence of infant resuscitation. Labor and delivery represent one of several situations where excessive medication is unquestionably dangerous. Finally,

Melzack (1970 a) states that there are many painful conditions that cannot be satisfactorily controlled by analgesics, local anesthetics or even neurosurgery. Regrettably, certain pain relief methods such as hypnosis, suggestion, relaxation and others historically have been suspect. He feels that greater attention to these methods will be beneficial for patients with pain. Therefore, we embark upon a discussion of many nursing activities, including the administration of analgesics, that may assist a patient with his pain experience.

Establishing a relationship with the patient with pain. When the patient has his first contact with a nurse, the foundation begins to be laid for dealing with any problems the patient may have. The nurse-patient relationship established at this time is particularly important when pain must be handled. A person may anticipate pain from the moment he becomes a patient, although he may not know the exact form of that pain. Whether the patient is in the anticipation, presence or aftermath phases of pain, his relationship with his nurse is significant. All of the activities the nurse performs with the patient establish her relationship with him, but here we are concerned with some of what often transpires in the initial contacts between the nurse and the patient with pain.

The patient's responses to his pain experience are a form of interpersonal communication. The nurse must indicate that she has received this message by communicating something to the patient. Not every patient automatically assumes that the nurse is concerned about him; that she can be trusted to help him and to believe him; that she wants to comply, if possible, with his expectations of her and of his total medical management; and that she can help him with the emotional and intellectual aspects of his pain experience as well as the physical aspects. Throughout the nurse-patient relationship it is the nurse's responsibility to establish such confidence.

Since establishing a relationship with the patient with pain begins during the first interactions with the patient, this nursing activity for pain relief necessarily overlaps with assessment. The manner in which the nurse obtains information about the patient communicates much to the patient about the potential nature of his relationship with her. The patient's perception of the nurse's intentions and trustworthiness probably significantly influences the effectiveness of all nursing activities for pain relief. During assessment the nurse can attempt to obtain the patient's trust and convey her concern for him. She may do this by maintaining the essential characteristics of what Szasz calls the "one-person situation" as opposed to the "two-person situation."

One- and two-person situations. In the one-person situation the patient is the only person involved. He does not communicate his feelings about his pain experience to anyone but himself. This means that the patient both experiences and observes his own pain and, therefore, the question of validating pain does not arise. In the one-person situation the patient does not risk disagreement between what he experiences and what another person may observe or believe.

In the two-person situation the patient communicates his pain to someone else. He risks disagreement once he has told another person about his pain. He exposes himself to the possibility that the other person may not believe him or may not interpret the pain experience as he does.

The nurse should attempt to maintain the qualities of the one-person situation by conveying that she believes the patient and is trying to understand how the patient experiences the pain (McCaffery and Moss). Mrs. Smith's interactions with her husband and her labor room nurse demonstrate how the nurse established a two-person situation and the husband a one-person situation. When Mrs. Smith was admitted she was dilated 2 cm. and had been in labor for 21 hours. The physician diagnosed her slow progress in labor as hypertonic uterine dysfunction and administered a barbiturate. This medication was supposed to stop the abnormal and unusually painful contractions and provide the needed rest until labor resumed. Since this was at midnight, the physician left and the nurse was responsible for observing the patient. The nurse turned out the overhead light, told the patient to try to rest, and then left. The husband turned on a small table lamp and continued to time the contractions at his wife's request. About two hours later Mrs. Smith called the nurse and said, "I don't think the medicine is working. I'm still having contractions and they're rather painful." The nurse felt the patient's uterus for a few minutes and replied, "You're not in labor. You just feel the baby kicking. Now let's turn out the light and you try to get some rest." The patient had communicated her pain to someone else and had risked disagreement with that person. The nurse established the two-person situation when she communicated her disagreement with the patient. In stating that labor had ceased the nurse implied that the patient was over-reacting to the baby's movements. Also, she did not offer any pain relief measures. The husband maintained the one-person situation by continuing to time what his wife continued to call contractions. Needless to say, Mrs. Smith did not summon the nurse again. Six hours later, when Mrs. Smith's physician arrived, he found her dilated to 6 cm. Mrs. Smith said to him, "I simply can't go on. The pain is too much."

In this situation, the nature of the nurse's error was that she did not believe the patient experienced pain. The nurse based her belief on not being able to determine an adequate physiological stimulus for pain. As a result she prolonged the patient's pain. In this particular case she dangerously delayed further medical intervention.

After delivery another nurse talked with Mrs. Smith about her labor. Mrs. Smith focused mostly on the pain she experienced during the night of her labor. When the nurse asked why she did not call the labor room nurse again, Mrs. Smith replied, "But she didn't believe I had pain." This statement reflects Mrs. Smith's awareness of the two-person situation and demonstrates how it destroyed her belief that the nurse was concerned and could be trusted. Later Mrs. Smith said that her husband believed she was in pain, and the nurse asked how she knew this was true. Mrs. Smith said, "Because he listened to what I said. As tired as he was he kept timing the contractions and rubbing my back." The husband maintained the essential characteristics of the one-person situation simply by acting in accordance with his wife's point of view. Mrs. Smith did not remember what he said, if anything, but his actions conveyed that he believed her and was concerned.

Nursing activities to relieve pain convey this same trustworthiness and concern, but the nurse's words may also transmit this message. For example, in addition to providing pain relief measures, the labor room nurse caring for Mrs. Smith could have said any one or several of the following: "What do the contractions feel like? Show me where you feel the discomfort. How often do the contractions occur? I'll keep my hand on your uterus for a while and you tell me when you feel a strong contraction." Not only would the nurse have obtained very important information, but she would have conveyed to Mrs. Smith a respect for what she was experiencing. The nurse's failure to feel a contraction need not have been used to invalidate Mrs. Smith's pain complaint. The nurse could have explored other causes of the discomfort and eventually considered that the dysfunctional labor was continuing.

When the nurse checks to discover the source of painful stimuli she must be careful not to let negative findings suggest to the patient that she does not believe he has pain. She can avoid this suggestion by obtaining a full description of the pain, by exploring the meaning of the pain to the patient, by offering pain relief measures, and by contacting the physician when indicated. In some emergency situations there is little time for the nurse to engage in a dialogue of this length with the patient. Nevertheless, she can establish eye contact and say something to the effect of, "The doctor and I are helping you as fast as we can." Among other things this conveys to the patient that his painful condition is recognized.

Eye contact. Establishing eye contact with a patient is especially important whenever the patient cannot or will not discuss his pain with the nurse. This lack of discussion of pain occurs not only in emergency situations but also when there is a language barrier, when the patient does not trust the nurse, when the patient is very fatigued, or when the patient is a child. Eye contact helps to convey that the nurse is concerned about the patient as an individual. One Negro patient was aware that many of the other Negro patients on the ward did not trust the white nurse enough to communicate their pain to her. He finally told her that she should make a greater effort to "look them in the eyes."

Play. Words are not always a good means of communicating with a young child. Other methods in addition to eye contact must be used to establish the nurse-child relationship. Conveying concern to the child and obtaining his trust often can be accomplished through the use of play. Even on a busy day for the nurse she can take the child to the playroom or provide him with toys. While she is giving him physical care the nurse can sing to him, recite nursery rhymes or television commercials, or make a game out of his bath. A short time after the nurse has been involved in some painful activity with the child, she should see him again. She can engage in some pleasant experience with him such as eating, playing or going for a walk. These types of interactions help the child understand that the pain he experiences as a result of the nurse's actions is not necessarily a hostile act on her part. And, he will be less prone to anticipate pain fearfully every time he sees the nurse if his interactions with the nurse encompass not only pain but happy times.

Compliance with the patient's expectations. Complying with the patient's expectations of his total medical care is another means of establishing a relationship with the patient and increasing his tendency to obtain pain relief. If the patient with pain receives the type of medical care he expects and values, he is likely to have less anxiety about his pain. Consequently he will have a greater tolerance for pain or experience a lower intensity of pain. Because of the patient's culture, for example, he may place more value on the personality of the nurse and physician than on their technical skill. With such a patient the nurse is probably more effective in assisting the patient with his pain experience if she establishes a relationship that includes social interactions. Traditionally the nurse has been admonished to maintain a "professional" relationship with the patient that minimizes attention to the nurse as an individual. While it is seldom helpful for the nurse to share her personal problems with the patient, many patients establish a more trusting relationship with the nurse if she shares something of her life such as her hobbies or the antics of her children. Naturally the nurse should not use this type of social interaction to avoid what the patient wants or needs to discuss.

Another patient such as one from the Jewish culture may value care that is focused on a cure for the cause of his pain. For this patient the nurse can explain all procedures and treatments in the context of how they contribute to determining the cause, controlling the cause or effecting a cure. Some pain relief measures can be explained in this way, promoting the patient's acceptance of pain relief. The patient who is concerned primarily with a cure for the cause of pain may be reluctant to accept any pain relief measure, especially an analgesic, if it is not a cure. In some cases the analgesic's contribution to a cure can be explained. For example, the patient suffering from painful muscle spasms associated with a ruptured intervertebral disc might be told, "Your discomfort is from muscle spasms. The more pain you have the more tense your muscles become and the greater the spasm. While this medication does not repair the disc, it relieves the pain which in turn reduces the spasm so that the disc can heal better." This statement demonstrates that the nurse is attempting to comply with the patient's expectations of his medical management. She stresses how the pain relief she offers is in accordance with the value the patient places on a cure.

Still another patient, such as one from the Old American culture, may tend to have greater confidence in his medical care if a large number of tests, treatments and medications are utilized, regardless of their purpose. With this patient the nurse can emphasize and discuss the various types of care he is receiving. She might even go so far as to place all his 10:00 a.m. medications in separate medicine cups. She could give them to him one at a time, thus emphasizing the number of pills he is receiving.

Within the context of compliance with what the patient values and expects in his total medical care, the nurse relates to the patient in other ways. She attempts to establish a relationship in which the patient knows that the nurse is willing and able to assist him with many of the emotional, intellectual and physical aspects of pain. Of course, the need to deal with these aspects of pain will vary between patients and within the same patient from one time to the next. But the nurse should demonstrate her concern for and ability to identify and deal with these aspects of pain. One way of doing this is by exploring with the patient the meaning of his pain experience.

Exploration of pain experience. The patient's anxiety during the period of anticipation of a painful procedure such as a pneumoencephalogram may be as much related to the possible pathological findings as it is to the impending discomfort. He may need to discuss the meaning of this painful procedure (emotional aspect) as well as the nature of the pain (intellectual aspect). Or, the patient's complaint of pain may be very far removed from what is actually bothering him. Nursing research has demonstrated that the nurse's exploration of the patient's request for pain relief may reveal that the patient needs information about his condition or self-care (intellectual aspect), that his visitors have upset him (emotional aspect), that he needs to empty his bladder (physical aspect), or that he needs to talk about his feelings with regard to being ill, alone or inactive (emotional aspect) (Bochnak, Rhymes and Leonard; McBride, 1967).

When the nurse's exploration of the meaning of pain to the patient reveals intellectual, emotional and/or physical needs, she has performed both assessment and intervention activities. In relation to assessment she has identified the meaning of pain to the patient. She can use this to determine appropriate intervention. If she discovers a physical need she may proceed to select an appropriate nursing activity such as administering a pharmacological agent. If an intellectual need is revealed she may consider nursing activities such as giving information or using the patient group situation. If the patient has an emotional need she may choose the nursing activities of remaining with the patient or utilizing other professional help.

Exploring the meaning of pain contributes to the nurse-patient relationship because it results in individualized care. This type of care helps to convince the patient of the nurse's concern and trustworthiness. Exploring the meaning of pain to the patient also clarifies the nurse's role. The patient becomes aware that the nurse intends to assist him with all aspects of his pain experience. Consequently, the patient's relationship with the nurse is based on an awareness of the nurse's concern and an understanding of the nurse's role. When this type of nurse-patient relationship exists, the effectiveness of all pain relief measures is increased. The findings of one study suggest that even when a pain relief measure is appropriate to the patient's needs, its effectiveness will be enhanced significantly if the meaning of pain is explored (McBride, 1967). For example, if a back rub is an appropriate pain relief measure for a particular patient, the back rub will result in greater pain relief if the nurse explores the meaning of pain to the patient.

Sometimes exploration of the meaning of pain to the patient is in itself sufficient intervention for pain relief. The mere opportunity for the patient to talk with someone about the meaning of his pain may serve to decrease fear, anxiety or depression. Or, exploration of the meaning of pain may facilitate the process of grief and mourning. The meaning of the patient's pain may be related to a number of things. The patient may fear unbearable pain and consequent loss of control. He may be depressed because pain prevents him from enjoying certain aspects of life. The patient may be in the process of grief and mourning over a permanent loss. Pain may cause him to fear for his life or remind him of a change in his body image or role. Or the patient may be anxious over his own irritability when he is in pain. He may fear the impact pain may have on his personality and interpersonal relationships. One nursing study found that one third of the patients were aware of and concerned about the relationship between their pain and its psychological effects. Some of these patients remarked that the pain made them irritable, crazy or prone to say things they did not mean (McBride, 1969).

Many studies indicate the importance of reducing the affects associated with pain, especially anxiety. As mentioned in Chapter 2, pain occurring in the absence of anxiety produces physiological responses comparable to those occurring in the orienting reaction to any novel stimulus. These responses may involve only slight increases in heart rate, in depth of respiration and in palmar sweating (Shor). The pain relief achieved through the reduction of anxiety is also observable in the patient's verbalizations, movements and other behaviors (Sternbach, 1968). Therefore, the nurse-patient relationship should include exploring the meaning of pain to the patient. This exploration may alleviate the emotions associated with the pain experience. Reduction in anxiety and other feelings will result in pain relief. Obviously, the exploration of the meaning of pain is only one of several nursing activities that may reduce anxiety or other affects. Any nursing activity that reduces affects associated with pain will produce pain relief.

When the nurse explores the meaning of pain to the patient she is assisting him to recognize and handle his feelings. Talking about these feelings encourages the patient to think about them and is the first step toward the patient's being able to determine a method of dealing with them. An example of this is the nurse's interaction with Mrs. Felton, who was admitted for an elective appendectomy. Mrs. Felton had anticipated being in the hospital for a few days and returning to work within three weeks. However, she developed a wound infection. At the time of this interaction she had been in the hospital ten days and in isolation for seven days. When the nurse answered the call light, Mrs. Felton said, "I think I'd like to have something for pain." The nurse replied, "Of course. Tell me about your pain." Mrs. Felton answered, "Well, the infection bothers me and I just ache all over." This remark offered two clues to the nurse—that the infection and not the pain was a source of concern and that generalized aching could be a sign of anxiety.

The nurse proceded with, "I imagine it's hard to lie here with an infection, all alone and uncomfortable." The patient replied, "Yes, it is. I never dreamed I'd still be here. I thought I'd be going back to work soon and now I don't know when." The nurse continued, "Thinking about not going back to work must be as bad as the pain and even make the pain worse?" Mrs. Felton answered, "That's true. Every time it hurts I think it's that much longer before I get to go back to work. I don't know what we're going to do." The nurse asked, "You mean financially?" When the patient nodded affirmatively, the nurse continued, "What have you and your husband considered about this?"

Mrs. Felton replied, "I guess that's the real problem. I can't talk to him about it. He doesn't want me to worry, and I can't mention the pain without thinking *he* will worry. And when he's here and the pain is bad, I just get cranky and then things are a mess." Mrs. Felton began to sob at this point and the nurse remained with her. The nurse continued to discuss the meaning of the patient's pain, that is, the anxiety over the inability to resume her role of working and earning money and her inability to communicate with her husband. At the end of the interaction Mrs. Felton had decided on some ways to handle her problems. She had decided to take an analgesic prior to her husband's visit so that the pain would not make her "cranky." She also intended to mention to her husband that now might be a good time to sell the antique furniture she had recently inherited from a distant relative and stored in the garage. Upon questioning she said she did not need the analgesic and thought she might take a nap. As a result of this interaction Mrs. Felton identified some of her problems and made plans to handle them. This appeared to relieve her anxiety and thereby relieve her pain. In addition, this exploration of the meaning of pain established a relationship between Mrs. Felton and the nurse. For the remainder of her hospitalization Mrs. Felton often initiated conversation with this nurse in an attempt to deal with her anxieties.

In another situation a similar type of interaction between the nurse and Mr. Glass revealed that this patient's increasing arthritic pain caused him to be depressed over the loss of his ability to play tennis. Mr. Glass was a bachelor and for many years his social life had consisted of playing tennis at a particular club. He played regularly on three nights and during the day every weekend. Over a period of about ten days the nurse helped Mr. Glass through the process of grief and mourning. At the beginning she pursued any mention Mr. Glass made of his loss. Toward the end she assisted him with a substitute for his loss. Apparently he did not feel comfortable with the idea of sitting around the club conversing with his friends. He needed some activity through which to relate to them. Chess was another favorite pastime at the club, and Mr. Glass began to mention that he wished he knew how to play chess. The nurse obtained books about chess from the hospital library, and Mr. Glass began to study them. At this point Mr. Glass began to request fewer analgesics, even when he was not reading his books and in spite of the fact that no physical findings indicated that the arthritic condition had improved. Through the nurse's attempts to explore the meaning of his pain, Mr. Glass, like Mrs. Felton, began to identify his problem and determine a method of handling it. This in turn contributed to pain relief.

With a young child, the nurse can explore the meaning of pain in another way. Even if a child has considerable facility with language, he often has difficulty identifying or admitting his feelings about pain. When a child seems unable to discuss his feelings about pain, the meaning of pain sometimes can be explored through projection. Projection is a frequent defense mechanism for the child. Hence, he may be encouraged to tell the nurse about the pain experience of another child. Or he may make up a story about a doll or some pictures of a child in the hospital. He may express his own feelings by attributing them to someone else.

A younger child without facility with language may be encouraged to use dolls to dramatize the meaning of his pain experience. This technique was tried with Howie, a five-year-old boy with leukemia who had daily finger pricks. He identified the laboratory technician who performed this as the "lab lady." She usually arrived early in the morning, shortly after he had awakened and long before his mother arrived. Howie would begin to cry loudly when he saw her and tried many means of escaping from her. He required restraint during the procedure. Afterwards he often yelled, "You're a mean lab lady," and continued to cry for as long as five minutes. One day following the finger prick the nurse gave him a doll and a tiny, blunt shiny object. She told him the doll was the "lab lady" and he could prick her finger. The first two days Howie vigorously poked the doll's entire body and yelled, "You're mean," and "Bad lab lady." By the fifth day Howie was poking only the doll's finger and saying, "Got to do this." Then he would hold the doll in his arms. He now cried only at the time his finger was actually pricked, and afterwards he reached for the nurse and cuddled in her lap for a few minutes. Play with the doll revealed the hostility with which he felt the laboratory technician performed the procedure and the hostility he felt toward her. Through the doll play he not only identified the anxiety associated with the hostile meaning he attributed to the painful event, but eventually he handled this hostility. He replaced hostility with the recognition that the procedure had to be performed and was not a hostile attack. He also identified his need for physical closeness afterwards, and the nurse responded appropriately. Thus, to the extent possible, the nurse established a relationship with Howie that allowed him to express freely the meaning of pain and to ask for help in handling it.

Using doll play to put a child in the role of a person who performs activities he cannot understand frequently decreases the child's misunderstanding. Play helps him learn something about the role of the person who hurt him. And, through play his anxiety decreases because he is given an opportunity to express it. Often he identifies what he needs to help him handle the situation, such as the need to be held.

Respect for the patient's response. Another significant aspect of establishing a relationship with the patient is to convey respect for the patient's behavioral responses to pain. The patient may be ashamed of his responses to pain, or he may fear that his responses will be unacceptable to others. The patient's evaluation of his own behavioral responses to pain may cause more anxiety than the pain itself. One study found that greater anxiety resulted from the threat of failing to live up to someone else's expectations than from the threat of pain (Hodges). Anxiety, of course, may contribute to an increased perception of pain. Therefore, it is important for the nurse to help the patient accept his own behavioral responses to pain. The nurse may accomplish this by praising the patient for his attempts to cope with pain. This conveys to the patient that he is behaving in an acceptable fashion. Regardless of how the child or adult patient expresses pain, the nurse may say, "I know this is very difficult for you. You're handling it well." If the patient is controlling his behavior but is expending a great amount of energy in trying not to cry or scream, the nurse may add, "But many people need to cry or scream from time to time. If you need to do this, then go ahead. I understand." This does not preclude the possibility of the nurse's teaching the patient other responses to pain such as relaxation. However, it is important to alleviate the anxiety that may arise when the patient finds his pain responses unacceptable to himself or to others.

Occasionally the nurse must accept the fact that the desired relationship with the patient is unlikely to develop. This may occur with the child who manifests a prolonged period of protest and despair over separation from his mother and who has experienced frequent and intense pain for a long time. An adult from a deprived minority group may be suspicious of a nurse from the dominant group. Another patient may ascribe a role to the nurse similar to that of a hotel maid. Whenever the nurse is unable to establish a relationship in which the patient is confident of her concern and trustworthiness and able to explore the meaning of his pain, she can make every effort to promote the desired relationship between the patient and someone else. With the child she may be able to arrange for the mother to visit more often. For the patient from a minority group she may be able to utilize other members of the health team having a similar background. When the patient ascribes a constricted role to the nurse, she may be able to get the physician to have more frequent contacts with the patient.

Teaching the patient about pain. The patient's understanding and retention of information about his pain experience may contribute to pain relief through reducing anxiety and other affects associated with pain. When anxiety is present there is a tendency for the patient to perceive a greater intensity of pain, which in turn increases anxiety. This produces a spiraling process in which the patient experiences greater and greater pain. This process can be interrupted by reducing or controlling anxiety. One way to reduce this anxiety is by helping the patient obtain accurate information about his pain experience. Teaching the patient about pain may alleviate anxiety in several ways. It may prevent the patient from using fear-producing fantasies to compensate for a lack of knowledge. It may focus his attention on ways he can participate in activities that help control to some extent both his pain and his care. It may facilitate communication between the patient and his physician or other health team members. And, it may reduce the element of surprise that may cause the patient to feel victimized.

The value of teaching the patient about pain has been suggested by the findings of a nursing study of over 300 surgical patients. Extensive preoperative preparation was given to 181 patients and omitted for 140 patients. This preparation included items that will be discussed in this section, such as postoperative exercises, the nature of the pain and pain-relief measures. Comparison of the two groups revealed that the group of patients who received preparation began oral narcotics earlier and were discharged from the hospital sooner (Healy). Adequate teaching, then, appears to decrease the intensity and duration of pain and to contribute to faster recovery.

What, how and when the nurse teaches the patient about pain depends upon her assessment of the patient's pattern of handling pain and her assessment of the factors that influence the patient's responses to the pain experience. The nurse must also know the nature of the pain involved, which phases of the pain experience will be present, and the possible pain relief measures available or to be used. The nurse will utilize all this knowledge to individualize the teaching plan for each particular patient. Following is a discussion of specific types of information the nurse may consider, including the various teaching methods she may employ and suggestions for when she should teach the patient.

Occurrence of pain. The most basic piece of information the patient must have is the fact that pain may occur. The nurse may describe to the patient a painful procedure that is unfamiliar to him. Unless the nurse mentions pain, it is quite possible for the patient to remain unaware that pain may be present. An explanation of a tubal insufflation, for example, does not necessarily prepare the patient for possible discomfort both during and after the procedure. It may be necessary to mention the discomfort because to the layman the injection of air may not suggest the possibility of pain. On the other hand, the patient may fear pain when none is likely. For instance, the patient unfamiliar with an electrocardiogram may anticipate electric shock. The probable presence or absence of pain should always be clarified for the patient. In the absence of a noxious stimulus the patient may feel pain if he expects it.

Simply knowing that pain may occur is particularly beneficial to the patient who values minimal responses to pain. If pain takes him by surprise he is less able to control such reflexive responses as "oh" or jerking away. This type of patient is likely to become anxious if he responds in this way.

Once the patient knows that pain may occur, he requires some specific information about it. Studies suggest that anxiety is reduced if he knows when the painful event will occur and how long the discomfort will last (Jones, Bentler and Petry). Using the patient who is to have a cholecystectomy, for example, the nurse may say, "The removal of your gall bladder is scheduled for 8 o'clock Tuesday morning, tomorrow morning. You probably will not be aware of any discomfort until about the middle of Tuesday afternoon. You will begin to wake up from the anesthetic at that time. You may be aware of discomfort in the area of the operation and perhaps of a sore throat. The discomfort you may feel probably will be the greatest during the first 24 hours. By Wednesday afternoon you will notice that it is lessening gradually and by Thursday afternoon you will feel more comfortable." Naturally this is only one of many types of information the nurse will give this patient. But this statement illustrates how a patient can be told when he may begin to experience the greatest discomfort and how long this will last. Further instruction would include such items as how long the milder pain would last and when the nasogastric tube would be removed.

Variety of sensations. The patient also needs to know the quality of all pain sensations and the possible variations in the quality. For example, the steady wound pain postoperatively may vary in both quality and intensity depending upon whether the patient is lying still, taking deep breaths or ambulating. In addition to the wound pain, the patient may experience discomfort from tubes inserted in other areas of the body, immobilization of a limb, venipuncture or injections. Through her readings the nurse can obtain information about the quality of the pain involved in various diagnostic and therapeutic procedures. Patients who have had these painful experiences may also provide information, perhaps more accurately and in greater detail.

In describing the quality of a pain sensation, the term "pain" probably should be avoided. To most patients, the word pain seems to suggest an almost intolerable sensation. Pain is also a rather general term that encompasses a variety of different sensations. When a general term is appropriate to use, the nurse may choose the words "uncomfortable," "discomfort" or "hurt." She may further qualify the terms with the adjectives "mild," "moderate," "considerable," "great" or "severe." Whenever possible the nurse should describe more precisely the discomfort with such terms as "pulling," "pressure," "aching," "contraction" or "stinging." The words "burning" and "pricking" may have a more ominous connotation, but sometimes an accurate description of discomfort requires their usage. The nurse may augment her description of the quality of the pain by demonstrating the sensation to the patient. Using his arm or leg, or better yet the actual site of future pain, she can pull or pinch the tissues or apply pressure. She can tell the patient this sensation is similar to the discomfort he may experience. This is a particularly important method of teaching the child who is not likely to understand or retain verbal instruction.

When the nurse is teaching the patient about the quality of the pain sensation, she should try to avoid presenting this information in a way that persuades the patient that he must or will have pain, especially severe pain. For example, while the nurse is demonstrating the pulling sensation the patient may feel at the site of the incision when he moves, she can say, "This is the kind of pulling sensation and discomfort you'll probably feel the first time you walk after your operation, except the discomfort may be greater than this." The nurse can make liberal use of the terms "may," "probably" and "possibly" rather than making flat statements such as "All patients feel uncomfortable," or "You will feel extremely uncomfortable." While some procedures seem to cause pain in most patients, there is always the possibility that this patient will be an exception. We have already noted that not all postoperative patients complain of pain, that some soldiers do not experience pain from severe combat wounds, and that any one of several factors may decrease the perceived intensity of pain. In addition to this, the nurse will be teaching the patient about pain relief measures. She does not want to persuade the patient to feel intense pain in spite of these measures.

This does not mean that the patient should never be told to expect severe discomfort. After the nurse has observed the patient's responses to various noxious stimuli, she may be able to make accurate predictions about his perception of the intensity of pain. The nurse may also be able to make these predictions on the basis of what the patient tells her about his past painful experiences. If she is reasonably certain that the patient will feel severe discomfort, it seems unfair to the patient not to prepare him for this. The nurse may still wish to qualify her remark by saying, "I may be wrong but I think you may find this very uncomfortable." One nursing study of 47 patients who had recently had open heart surgery revealed that about 70 percent were satisfied with their preoperative instruction. However, a few suggested that the patient should be told more about the severity of the pain since they experienced a greater level of pain than they were led to expect (Jarvis).

When the nurse teaches the patient about the quality of the pain sensation he may experience, she includes information about the location of the pain. Pain may occur in an area of the body that the patient views as a socially unacceptable topic of conversation. It is important for the nurse to teach the patient terminology for that area of the body, and use it often so that the patient becomes more comfortable with its usage. Especially when pain occurs in the urethra, rectum, vagina or scrotum, medical terminology often seems more appropriate and acceptable to the patient than the terms laymen tend to employ. Following a hemorrhoidectomy, one patient was lying in bed in obvious distress. He responded to the nurse's questions with incomplete sentences, hesitation and avoidance of eye contact. Finally he blurted out, "The manure is gonna come out for the first time." This man, from a rural area in Tennessee, could find no more appropriate terminology to describe a situation that embarrassed him. The nurse could have assisted him by acquainting him with the term "bowel movement" or "BM." This might have decreased his embarrassment and increased the likelihood of his asking for pain relief measures.

Allay the patient's fears about personal safety. Another aspect of teaching the patient about pain concerns the safety of his experience. The patient may fear that his pain will escalate and be beyond anyone's control or that his pain is indicative of untoward effects or complications. If he thinks either of these things, he will be less able to tolerate the pain and/or will perceive a greater intensity of pain (Bronzo and Powers). Anxiety increases when the patient believes his situation is unsafe. Telling the patient what types of uncomfortable sensations he may experience and when these may occur helps to alleviate this source of anxiety. When the patient feels them, he will not tend to suspect that something has gone wrong. In addition, teaching the patient about pain relief measures will help to assure him that his pain will not be uncontrolled. Further, the nurse can stress that the patient's condition will be monitored closely and that the people involved in his care are quite competent. This is especially important when ethics require that the physician tell the patient the risks involved in a procedure. In such cases it is helpful to the patient if the nurse can say honestly, "You are in very good hands with Dr. — — — —. He knows as much or more than anyone else about this." Even when the risks are minimal and virtually unmentioned to the patient, it is always possible that the patient has some preconceived ideas about the possible complications of his situation. For example, the patient may have the unrealistic fear of permanent back injury from a spinal anesthetic. When the nurse's assessment has been comprehensive, she will have discovered these misconceptions and can correct them.

The source of a young child's feelings about a lack of safety is often associated with being deprived of his parents. The young child tends toward artificialism, or regarding things as being under the almost complete control of human beings. This means that the presence of his mother may be very reassuring to him. Because his mother has cared for him in the past, the child will tend to regard her, and not the nurse, as the expert. The nurse may relieve a great deal of the child's anxiety if she says, for example, "When you return to this room your mother will be here." Since the young child may not fully understand verbal explanation, the best thing the nurse can do to increase his sense of safety is to allow the mother to be present as much as possible.

Another method of increasing the patient's feeling of safety and of eliminating possible sources of anxiety is to acquaint the patient in advance with all the personnel, procedures, rooms and objects he is likely to encounter during all phases of his pain experience. This will decrease his anxiety and thereby increase his ability to cope with pain. With the advent of television and the current popularity of medical dramas, the general public fortunately has become more informed about the physical appearance of hospital personnel, mechanical devices, operating rooms, and so on. The patient still should be told to which of these he will be exposed. He also needs to become familiar with and understand the purposes of the procedures and equipment pertaining to his care. Regardless of whether or not the procedures and equipment will actually cause pain, their strangeness may arouse anxiety and thereby contribute to pain. With regard to those activities that both cause pain and require the patient's cooperation and participation, knowledge of the purpose of the activity is especially important. When the patient knows that something painful contributes to his well-being, he is more willing to cooperate and better able to tolerate the pain.

Use many sensory modalities to teach the patient. The teaching method that maximizes understanding uses many of the patient's sensory modalities. This means that in addition to whatever verbal instruction is appropriate, the patient sees, handles, hears and participates tactilely and kinesthetically. Both children and adults should have an opportunity at least to see equipment before it is used in conjunction with a painful event. Children should be encouraged to touch and handle the equipment. If the patient is to have surgery this equipment might include the cardiac monitor, an oxygen tent, and equipment used with intravenous fluids, closed chest drainage, or endotrachial suctioning. It is important, too, for the patient to hear the sounds associated with suctioning, monitors and other noisy equipment. The nurse should also rehearse with the patient such activities as coughing, turning, and getting in and out of bed. She should explain to the adult and older child that these help prevent "gas pains," pneumonia and blood clots. In the author's personal experience with the child undergoing surgery, postoperatively the child is remarkably tolerant and calm about events, including pain, if he has been acquainted with them preoperatively.

And by contrast, the same child is surprisingly anxious about seemingly more simple events such as rectal temperatures or vomiting when he has not been warned of their possible occurrence.

The principle of using many sensory modalities to teach the patient about pain applies to children and adults, but with the young child its application is almost mandatory. We have seen that words usually are not reliable symbols of communication with a child below the age of seven years, although he may manifest great facility with language. In support of this, the findings of one study suggest that the child obtains more correct reflections of reality from practical manipulation of objects than he does from merely touching and seeing objects (Zaporozhets). And Piaget contends that the child's thought becomes more logical as a result of interpersonal interactions in which the child is actually forced to recognize the roles of others. Further, study of the effects of verbal explanation alone as a method of preparation for surgery has shown that this is not as effective with children younger than four years as it is with children older than four years (Vaughn).

The use of many sensory modalities to teach the patient about pain can be illustrated by the preparation of a patient for the removal of sutures from a lower abdominal wound. A verbal explanation might be adequate for an adult patient. Allowing the adult to handle the equipment, such as the tweezers, scissors and suture, would probably render the procedure completely understandable to him. But, this type of explanation would be insufficient for the young child. It would be more consistent with his cognitive level if he were encouraged to manipulate these objects in their appropriate relation to one another. This could be accomplished by helping the child remove the sutures in a doll's abdomen. The child could watch the nurse demonstrate what would happen. Then he could participate tactilely and kinesthetically by removing a few of the doll's sutures (McCaffery, 1969). Also, the nurse could gently pull and pinch the skin on his upper abdomen, telling him this is what he might feel.

With an even younger child, below the age of two years, for example, there is little hope of his comprehending an event such as suture removal. Also, he may lack the motor ability to remove sutures from a doll. However, he can watch the nurse remove the doll's sutures and he can play with the equipment. This does not really explain much to a child this age, but it may decrease possible fear of strange equipment.

Teach the patient about pain relief. Teaching about pain should always include pain relief measures. The only exception is the patient who cannot comprehend even minimal verbal explanation accompanied by a demonstration. The child below the age of two years is usually one of these exceptions. All other patients should learn as much as possible about ways of relieving their pain.

Perhaps the first thing the patient should know is that the nurse considers that helping him achieve pain relief is one of her responsibilities. Therefore, at the beginning of a discussion on pain relief it may help the patient understand what he can expect from the nurse if she says, for example, "I want to help you stay as comfortable as possible, so let's talk about the many ways I can help you with this."

The possibility of pain relief is enhanced when teaching the patient about pain includes what the patient believes will relieve pain. Or, the nurse may provide information that convinces the patient of the effectiveness of certain pain relief measures. Pain relief is much more likely to occur if the patient believes in the effectiveness of the pain relief measure. This fact may be related to the mechanism of classical conditioning or to the resolution of cognitive dissonance.

Classical conditioning relates to the patient's belief in a pain relief measure in the following way. As a result of the patient's past experience with pain, a particular pain relief measure may have been paired with achieving pain relief often enough for the patient to be conditioned to experience pain relief. This pain relief will tend to occur regardless of whether or not there is any physiological basis for it. In the absence of actual experience with pain relief, the patient may be partially conditioned to expect it from certain measures if he physically or mentally rehearses the pain relief measure.

Pain relief from a measure the patient believes in may be related to the resolution of cognitive dissonance. This notion is derived from Festinger's theory that cognitive dissonance is a motivating state of affairs. Cognitive dissonance occurs, for example, when the individual's behavior is inconsistent with what he believes. This dissonance motivates him to change either his behavior or his belief. For instance, dissonance could occur if the patient believes that moist heat should relieve his pain, but he continues behavioral manifestations of pain when the moist heat is applied. His belief about moist heat is dissonant with his behavioral response to moist heat. Theoretically the patient then becomes motivated to resolve this dissonance through either of two possibilities. He may change his belief that moist heat relieves pain, or he may change his behavioral response and act as he would if he had experienced pain relief. Studies indicate that when the person resolves dissonance by behaving as if he experienced a lesser intensity of pain, both verbal and physiological responses are consistent with pain relief (Zimbardo, *et al.*). In other words, the patient is not "fooling" anybody. He actually perceives a decreased intensity of pain. Of course, not all patients will resolve their dissonance in this way. Some will tolerate dissonance, and others will change their beliefs about the effectiveness of the pain relief measure.

The nurse's assessment of the patient includes determining the patient's opinion about what, if anything, will relieve pain. Assessment also includes whether or not the patient has used any particular pain relief methods with success. Whenever possible the pain relief measures the patient believes in should be made available. Although aspirin is pharmacologically as potent as any non-prescription analgesic, it may not be as effective for the particular patient as the commercial preparation from which he previously has obtained pain relief. If the specific medication cannot be obtained through the hospital pharmacy, the nurse may be able to obtain the physician's approval to have the patient's own supply brought from his home.

Sometimes the pain relief measure favored by the patient is contraindicated. Nevertheless, the nurse can utilize this information. For example, any preparation containing aspirin may be too hazardous for the patient with hepatic disease or gastrointestinal irritation. However, the nurse can explain that an antacid relieves gastric discomfort more effectively than aspirin by coating and protecting the site of the injury. Or, the patient who has used the accelerated breathing patterns of the Lamaze method may have to be warned that this may increase her chest pain following thoracic surgery. However, the nurse can encourage this patient to use other aspects of the Lamaze method such as relaxation, concentration, and slow, rhythmic breathing.

In addition to utilizing those measures the patient believes will relieve pain, the nurse explains other pain relief measures that will probably be appropriate for the particular patient's pain experience. Various possible pain relief measures are discussed in the remainder of this chapter. Each one is accompanied by specific suggestions about how it may be explained to the patient, including telling the patient why the method relieves pain and what, if any, participation is required of him. Here we will consider important aspects of the nurse's approach to any pain relief measure. Certain statements and approaches may be used with all pain relief measures to promote their effectiveness.

Presenting the pain relief measure. Most pain relief measures are more effective when used before pain becomes intense. Some measures should be used in the period of anticipation of pain before any pain sensation is felt. Others should be applied when pain is of mild or moderate intensity, before pain becomes severe. The basic reason for early application of a pain relief measure is related in part to the control of anxiety. The sensation of pain, especially if it is severe, activates various sources of anxiety. Generally anxiety increases the perceived intensity of pain, causing more anxiety. Obviously this spiraling process is easier to control in the early stages than when the patient approaches the panic level. Therefore, the patient should be asked to report his pain to the nurse as soon as it begins or as soon as it increases in intensity. It is especially important to stress this to the patient from the lower socioeconomic class. Several studies suggest that persons from this group do not feel as free to request pain relief measures as do persons from the upper socioeconomic class (Bruegel; Loan and Morrison).

In the initial preparation of the patient for various pain relief measures he may utilize, the nurse should be sure the patient has realistic expectations of the duration and degree of pain relief that may be achieved. Very few pain therapies will completely eliminate the sensation of pain. Usually little discussion is necessary to insure that the patient is aware of the limits of pain relief measures. Often the nurse conveys this information by saying, for example, "You may still be aware of some discomfort but it will not be as great (or, will not bother you as much). You probably will have to do this each time you feel uncomfortable (or, will not need this more often than every four hours)."

When a pain relief measure is indicated, the nurse should encourage the patient to decide which of several possible ones he wishes to employ to alleviate his pain. The nurse engages the patient's active participation in making a decision about what will relieve his pain. One nursing study indicated that this approach often resulted in pain relief without the use of medication (Moss and Meyer). The nurse may ask the patient which measures he believes will alleviate his pain. The nurse may also explain measures that she believes will relieve pain. When the patient and the nurse have identified one possible pain relief measure, preferably several measures, the nurse may then say, "Would you like to try (*a specific measure*) now? Do you think this will relieve your discomfort?" When the patient responds affirmatively or is willing to try the measure, he has decided that he may or will obtain pain relief. That the patient has made this decision increases the probability that pain relief will result. If the patient does not want to try the pain relief measure, then the nurse may ask him about others until she finds one that the patient believes will be effective. In addition to the pain relief measures discussed in the remainder of the chapter, the nurse should remember that teaching the patient about the cause of pain sometimes provides pain relief. To involve the patient in a decision about this, the nurse might say, "Do you think your discomfort would bother you less if you knew what caused it?" Again, the patient is making a decision about what will relieve his pain.

Involving the patient in decision making about pain relief probably is an effective maneuver only if it is done in the context of the nurse-patient relationship described at the beginning of this chapter. Among other things, this decision making should be preceded by obtaining the patient's trust and conveying concern and by assisting the patient to describe his pain experience.

Immediately prior to the administration or use of any pain relief measure the nurse's positive suggestion of pain relief may increase the likelihood of pain relief. The nurse may say, for example, "I think this will help relieve your discomfort," or "This will certainly make you feel better." The idea that such a statement contributes to pain relief originated with the numerous placebo studies (e.g., Gliedman, *et al.*). In these studies many subjects obtained pain relief from placebos when they were told that the medication would undoubtedly relieve their pain. However, nursing research has shown that a positive statement about pain relief is not effective when it is used alone without other nurse-patient interaction (Chambers and Price). As with the use of decision making, the effectiveness of a positive statement about pain relief is dependent in part upon the quality of the relationship between the patient and the nurse.

Interestingly enough, a positive statement of pain relief tends to be less effective when it is accompanied by the suggestion that further action for pain relief will be taken if necessary (Billars). When the nurse assures the patient of further action if pain is not relieved, she implies that the present pain therapy may not be effective. This apparently undermines the positive suggestion of pain relief. Therefore, when a pain relief measure is about to be used by the patient, the nurse may enhance its effectiveness by omitting any suggestion of further action. The nurse tells the patient that the measure should relieve his discomfort, but she does not tell him that something else will be done if this particular measure fails. Of course, the nurse will take further action if the patient's pain is not alleviated. And the teaching the nurse does prior to administering a pain relief measure may still include telling the patient about a variety of available pain relief measures. Omitting the suggestion of further action to relieve pain seems to be important only after the patient makes a decision to employ a particular pain therapy for the discomfort he is experiencing at the moment.

When to begin teaching about pain? Except for those interactions that occur at the time a pain relief measure is utilized, the nurse must decide *when* to teach the patient about pain. In making this decision the nurse must consider the patient's condition, whether or not an intrusive procedure is involved, and when the pain will occur if it is not already present. Ideally the patient's condition should be one of relaxation, alertness and freedom from pain, distractions and interruptions. A certain amount of anxiety is also advantageous because it facilitates learning. These characteristics are more likely to be present during the anticipation of pain than during the presence of pain. Hence, much emphasis is placed upon preparing the patient for pain prior to its occurrence. The question then becomes: how far in advance should the patient be prepared?

As a rule, the nurse should begin teaching the patient about pain as soon as he is aware that he will experience pain. Even if it will be quite some time before pain will occur, some teaching should be done. For example, the patient is often told days or weeks in advance that he must be hospitalized for a painful treatment. This means that the nurse working in the physician's office, an outpatient clinic or a public health agency is frequently in a position to begin to prepare the patient for impending pain. If the painful event does not require hospitalization and will be done immediately on an outpatient basis, the nurse proceeds at once to teach the patient about pain in the comprehensive manner already discussed. But, when pain will occur later, in the hospital, the nurse in an outpatient setting begins the teaching process by discussing with the patient some aspects of his hospitalization. It is unrealistic to assume that the nurse in the outpatient setting can prepare the patient thoroughly several days in advance for all the painful situations he may encounter in the hospital. Besides the fact that some painful events are unknown prior to hospitalization, the patient may not retain the information. Also he may be more concerned with making arrangements for his absence from home or work. However, to control the patient's anxiety and to prevent him from engaging in frightening fantasies, the nurse can focus his attention on some elements of his future hospitalization. Many times the physician already has told the patient about a painful procedure that definitely will be performed. This information plus the nurse's assessment of what concerns the patient at the time enables her to select some events on which to focus the patient's attention. In addition, she may suggest that the patient call her if questions arise later.

The teaching the nurse can do on an outpatient basis is illustrated by the interaction between Mr. Barnes and his physician's office nurse. The nurse had heard the physician tell Mr. Barnes that his left inguinal herniorrhaphy was scheduled for a week from that day. The physician had also discussed financial aspects, length of hospitalization and activity restrictions following surgery. As Mr. Barnes was leaving the office the nurse asked him, "Would you like to sit down with me for a few minutes and discuss your operation?" Mr. Barnes sat and talked with the nurse for about ten minutes. His first comments pertained to the impact this surgery would have on his life style, particularly how long he would be unable to work, and the financial arrangements. The difference illness makes in the patient's usual way of living is typically the initial concern of the older child and adult. Helping the patient determine what to do about these problems prior to the illness alleviates a source of anxiety that may contribute to pain. Therefore, the nurse listened to the patient's plans and made a few additional suggestions the patient had not considered.

The nurse then asked Mr. Barnes if he were concerned about how he would feel the first few days after surgery. He replied, "I imagine I'll feel pretty rotten, but I'll live through it. Nothing I can do about that." Again, this patient's remark is rather typical. He anticipates pain and seems to feel powerless to do anything about it. Most patients are anxious about impending pain. However, they know so little about it they often ask very few questions. The most frequent question is that of asking for reassurance that analgesics will be available. Consequently, the nurse told Mr. Barnes that he could ask for medication to relieve his discomfort, and she also gave him information about another pain relief measure. Through a description and partial demonstration the nurse explained proper positioning, telling Mr. Barnes, "If you will keep your left leg bent in this way while you're lying in bed and when you move, you will help prevent discomfort from pulling and pressure on the repaired hernia. When you get ready for bed tonight, practice turning from side to side with your left leg bent." In purposely telling the patient about a pain relief measure that he could perform himself, and that he could practice prior to hospitalization, the nurse followed the principle that anxiety may be controlled by focusing the patient's attention on a specific aspect of the situation and by giving him something he can do. This patient will need to learn much more about pain when he enters the hospital. But, as soon as he was told when the painful event would occur, the office nurse began to contribute to the learning process about pain relief. She explored the meaning of his pain in terms of work and finances. She also taught him about two pain relief measures, analgesics and positioning.

Problems related to forewarning the patient of pain. Many painful situations are associated with intrusive procedures, such as injections, surgery and lumbar punctures. Intrusive procedures tend to be more anxiety-provoking than those procedures that do not invade the body such as exercise of a painful joint. When the patient is told about an intrusive procedure many hours or days in advance of its occurrence, he has time to engage in vivid fantasies about a horrible ordeal. For this reason it has been suggested that the patient be forewarned of an intrusive procedure only a short time before it is performed (Janis). This advice is often impossible to apply, in the case of surgery, for example. However, sometimes the nurse is able to elicit the physician's cooperation about when to tell the patient of an intrusive procedure. It may be the physician's practice to inform the patient about a procedure as soon as the physician decides it is indicated. This means, for example, that on a Monday morning the patient may be told he will have a lumbar puncture on Tuesday afternoon. The nurse may ask the physician to delay telling the patient until late Tuesday morning. This will allow ample time for teaching the patient, but it reduces the amount of time during which the patient may dread the event.

Regardless of whether or not the painful event is intrusive, the decision is sometimes made not to forewarn the patient of pain. The reason most frequently given for making this judgment is that the patient's knowledge of impending pain will cause him to become upset and worried. Undoubtedly this is usually true. Few patients remain undisturbed about the prospect of pain. But it is desirable for the patient to have a moderate level of anticipatory fear. One study of surgical patients showed that those with moderate anticipatory anxiety had a better postoperative adjustment than those with high or low anticipatory anxiety (Janis). Of course, if the patient is told only that he will experience pain, his anxiety may soar to undesirable heights. However, we have already mentioned that the patient should be taught much more than this about pain and that a discussion of pain relief measures should always be included. It would seem that if a patient is taught adequately about pain, he will be more able to cope with pain when it occurs. Therefore, in this author's opinion, the patient should always be forewarned of pain. Usually the forewarning should be sufficiently in advance to allow for adequate teaching, but there are two exceptions to this.

The first exception is the patient who is already being taught about a specific recurring, painful event but continues to manifest a considerable increase in anxiety when he is told exactly when the event will occur. He may even ask the nurse not to tell him. In a sense this type of patient has already been forewarned because he knows the painful event will recur at some time. Further, he is already being taught about his pain. While most patients benefit from knowing in advance exactly when pain will be felt, an occasional patient is highly anxious about his pain. The anxiety occurs in spite of the nurse's efforts to teach him, and he attempts to control his anxiety by denying or suppressing the fact that the painful event will occur again. The nurse's efforts to help him control his anxiety, such as teaching him about pain, should continue. However, he should not be warned that pain will occur in an hour or even several minutes. Warning of when pain will occur should be given only a few seconds in advance.

For example, this type of situation frequently occurs with the young child receiving injections every six hours. Among other activities for pain relief, the nurse may be teaching the child about injections by encouraging him to give injections to a doll. The child usually knows that he probably will receive other injections, but if he is very anxious about injections he may attempt to suppress this fact. It is rarely advisable to tell this child at ten o'clock in the morning that he will receive his next injection after lunch. However, when the nurse enters the room with the medication tray, the child is likely to know at once that he will receive an injection. At that point the nurse should tell him it is time for his injection. She should administer the injection as quickly as possible, shortening the time between forewarning and pain.

The second exception to forewarning the patient of pain minutes or hours in advance is a variation of the preceding one. This exception involves the patient who is exposed to a variety of different painful events, but the nurse observes that forewarning and teaching do not control his anxiety. Sometimes this patient too will ask the nurse not to tell him about impending pain. Or, he will perspire, vomit and manifest other signs of anxiety each time the nurse attempts to teach him about a future painful event. When this occurs, the nurse may try a different approach. Rather than telling the patient about the specific event and exactly when it will occur, she can teach him various pain relief measures such as rhythmic breathing and distraction. Then she can suggest that he practice these and use them whenever he feels uncomfortable. However, this patient too should be forewarned of pain in the second or two preceding the painful event.

When the nurse's assessment indicates the advisability of a very brief period of time between forewarning the patient of pain and the occurrence of pain, it is helpful if she discusses this with the patient, especially the adult patient. The nurse may tell the patient that he seems to be very anxious when he is warned of pain minutes or hours in advance. She may explore this with the patient and then involve him in making a decision about how he would like to handle this problem. She may say, for example, "You will be having other experiences that you may also find uncomfortable. Would you be less bothered by them if you were told about them at the very last second?"

Teaching during the presence of pain. If a patient is experiencing pain and has been taught little about it, he needs to learn about his pain and the available relief measures. The fact that the patient manifests severe pain should not prevent the nurse from attempting to teach him about pain. The nurse can pursue an interaction that includes the important elements of: telling the patient she wants to help him; asking for a description of the pain; exploring any clues as to the meaning of the pain to the patient; suggesting and explaining a pain relief measure and/or asking the patient what he thinks will relieve his pain; engaging him in making a decision about the effectiveness of a specific pain relief measure; and telling him the chosen measure will make him more comfortable. The nurse is often hesitant to initiate such an interaction with a patient who is in severe pain. She feels compelled to do something immediately to relieve the pain. But the nurse must remember that the interaction suggested above contains measures that produce or enhance pain relief. Whenever the patient responds to any part of this interaction with lack of interest, anger or impatience, the nurse simply proceeds to the next portion of the interaction. In other words, the nurse provides the patient with an opportunity to engage in this particular type of interaction, but she does not force him into it.

Sometimes the patient with pain demands a specific pain relief measure such as an analgesic and does not respond to the nurse's attempts at verbal interaction. In this situation the wisest course of action is probably to administer the analgesic. Once the patient has obtained what he desires, the nurse may then attempt the interaction again. Unless the analgesic is administered intravenously, 15 to 45 minutes may elapse before it is effective. The nurse may utilize this time to teach the patient about another pain relief measure, perhaps telling him that it will assist him until the analgesic becomes effective. Or, the nurse may attempt the interaction when the patient is experiencing less pain.

Using the patient group situation. Much of what a patient should know about pain need not be taught to him on a one-to-one tutorial basis. In fact, it can be taught as well or better to a group of patients. Teaching several patients about pain rather than teaching them individually has advantages for both the nurse and the patient. For the nurse, teaching a group means she can reach a larger number of patients in a shorter amount of time. For example, recent publications indicate that preoperative instruction on an individual basis requires a minimum of ten to 15 minutes of the nurse's time (Healy), but comparable instruction may be given to four patients in about 30 minutes (Mezzanotte). Teaching a group of patients is also likely to improve the organization, consistency and thoroughness of the nurse's instruction. Teaching materials, including the equipment with which the patient should become familiar, are assembled only once instead of several times for each patient.

When the plan for teaching a group of patients about pain includes an opportunity for group discussion, there are several advantages for the patient who is a member of the group. He may learn more, because group participation seems to stimulate a person to meet goals beyond those he would achieve if he were taught individually (Bonner). Also, the patient may find it reassuring to meet other patients who share the same problem of learning to cope with pain. This need to reduce the loneliness and uniqueness of having a particular health problem is testified to by the numerous clubs composed of patients with a common health problem. These organizations include such groups as Alcoholics Anonymous, colostomy clubs and Paralyzed Veterans of America. The exchange of ideas and sharing of solutions to problems is facilitated in groups like these because they meet regularly. Even if a group of patients being taught about pain meets only once, an opportunity to discuss the information presented may elicit some helpful comments and suggestions from group members. A group member may also benefit from questions asked by other members. Some questions may not have occurred to him or he may be hesitant to ask them. In addition, group discussion may influence a group member to change his opinion about his painful experience. This may be a significant advantage for the patient with either a high or low anticipatory fear of his impending painful experience.

There are several ways in which the nurse may utilize the group situation to produce the desired moderate level of anticipatory fear about pain. Research indicates that conformity to group opinion is more likely to occur when a large majority holds a contrary opinion and when that opinion must be made public (Hare). Therefore, the nurse may select the membership of the group to assure that the majority of patients will have moderate anticipatory fear. She can identify these patients on the basis of such behaviors as occasional restlessness, mild insomnia, and verbal admission of some concerns about the impending experience (Janis). In the group discussion the nurse can attempt to have each patient express the degree to which he is worried. This may influence the patient with high or low anxiety to change his opinion of the impending painful event. His anxiety may increase or decrease to the level manifested by the majority of patients. Even when the nurse cannot control the composition of the group she can utilize the other methods of promoting a moderate level of anticipatory anxiety. These methods include reinforcing the comments made by patients with moderate anxiety, making fear-arousing but realistic statements about the impending pain, and focusing on what the patient may do to achieve pain relief. When the nurse teaches an individual or a group about pain, she must remember that her goal is not to produce an unworried patient who calmly awaits his pain. It is necessary for the patient to worry about his pain so that he may find some ways of handling it.

We have discussed some of the advantages to both patient and nurse of the use of group teaching and have suggested some methods of capitalizing on the group process to achieve the desired advantages for the patient. We will now review some of the situations in which groups may be taught about pain. We will also consider some guidelines for determining the size of the group and a few of the ways the nurse may initiate and conduct a group.

Opportunities for group teaching. Teaching a group of patients about pain is an increasingly common practice. In the United States in the last decade, numerous groups of women with their husbands assembled on a regular basis during the last trimester of pregnancy to learn about the Read or the Lamaze method of comfortable labor and delivery. Mention has already been made of the encouraging results of preoperative instruction given to groups of adult patients in the hospital. In addition, some far-sighted nurses in Phoenix, Arizona, report that they have initiated programs in the schools and kindergartens to familiarize groups of children with hospital procedure, equipment and dress (Abbott, Hansen, and Lewis).

The opportunities for teaching people about pain in groups are almost limitless. When the nurse works in a setting where several patients each day need to be taught about impending but similar painful experiences, she may consider the possibility of teaching these patients in a group. For example, in an outpatient hematology clinic several patients may be taught about bone marrow aspiration. On a hospital cardiac unit more than one patient may need to learn about cardiac catheterization. Several patients recovering from myocardial infarctions may need to learn what to do in the event of another infarction. Several patients on a urological unit may be scheduled for cystoscopies on the same day. Even on the surgical unit of a small hospital, patients facing surgery the next day need to be taught many of the same things. In all of these situations the nurse may be able to reap the advantages of using the group situation to teach patients about pain.

Size of group. To teach patients about pain in a group, the ideal size of the group appears to be five, including the nurse. For example, the group might be composed of four patients and one nurse. In some cases it may be advisable to include a physician. Many times it is appropriate for the patient to bring a family member.

There are several reasons for suggesting that the group be five in number. Research on interpersonal relations in the small group reveals that in five-member groups individuals are more satisfied with the discussion and with the size of the group. The group is small enough to allow sufficient time for each member to contribute to the discussion. On the other hand, it is large enough to allow a member to withdraw comfortably from an awkward position without being pressured to expand upon it. In groups smaller than five members, there is an increased strain on each member to participate whether or not he wishes to contribute. A five-member group is also large enough to reduce the possibility that one person will be alone and unsupported in his opinion. This size group tends to split into a majority of three and a minority of two (Hare). This may be important during a discussion when a difference of opinion occurs over an issue that need not be resolved in a similar manner by everyone. Such an issue may be whether or not a family member should stay with the patient in pain.

Naturally, it is not always possible to have a group of five members but large groups should be avoided. If the nurse wishes to promote some discussion she may find it difficult with a group of over 20 members. Also, members of a group must take time to get to know each other at the beginning of a group meeting. This takes less time with fewer people. Further, members tend to be more self-conscious about participation in a very large group than they are in a small group. Therefore, whenever possible the nurse probably should attempt to keep the size of the group small.

Conducting a group. Most of the advantages to the patient of learning in a group depend on the group discussion. Therefore, the comments thus far have assumed that the majority of groups will utilize discussion either partially or exclusively. In some instances the patients in the group may possess sufficient knowledge to employ discussion only, obtaining additional information from each other as well as from the nurse. This may occur, for example, after the initial meeting of a group of cardiac patients that meets more than once to talk about how to handle another myocardial infarction. Or, it may occur in the first and only meeting of a group composed of patients who are having repeated skin grafts for burns. Even if there is only one meeting of the group and the nurse must present a certain amount of information as in preoperative instruction, time should be allotted for discussion.

Preoperative instruction can be utilized to illustrate how a nurse may be an effective leader in initiating and conducting a group for the purpose of teaching adult patients about pain. Since this group will meet only once and must learn some specific things, the nurse will keep the group small in number. And she will use a combination of lecture, demonstration and discussion. The material she teaches will consist mostly of those things all the patients need to know. The following is an example of the content and presentation method the nurse might use: verbal description, pictures or tour of the operating room or induction room and the recovery room or intensive care unit; verbal explanation of preoperative preparation such as clothing worn to the operating room, medications the night and morning prior to surgery, shaving the operative site, and removing valuables and teeth, including the reasons for these routines; verbal explanation of the location, quality and duration of various postoperative discomforts, asking each patient to demonstrate the quality and location of operative discomfort on himself by pulling the skin and applying pressure over the operative site; verbal explanations and demonstrations of pain relief measures such as medication, distraction and positioning; verbal explanation of policies regarding visitors, including the reasons for these rules; verbal explanation of the methods and purposes of deep breathing, coughing, leg exercises and turning, including a demonstration by the nurse and a brief practice session for the patients; showing, demonstrating and explaining the purposes of various equipment such as intravenous fluids, dressings, suction machines, cardiac monitors or any devices relevant to the majority of patients. Content might be added or deleted, depending upon the characteristics of the particular group of patients and the usual routines of the hospital. The nurse may also give each patient a printed sheet that emphasizes and summarizes the important parts of the content.

To encourage the patient to attend the group meeting, the nurse should approach him soon after his admission to the hospital. She should explain the nature of the group meeting, including the time, duration, place and purpose. The purpose of the meeting should not be stated in terms of teaching him about pain. The use of the term pain usually should be avoided. A better method of relating the purpose of the meeting is to explain how the activities of the group will meet some of the patient's needs such as information and socializing. To promote the cohesiveness of the group the nurse should also inform the patient of the similarity between himself and the other group members and suggest that he will get along well with the others. For example, the nurse may incorporate these ideas by saying to the patient, "I understand you are to have an operation tomorrow. Several other patients will be having operations tomorrow, too. Tonight at 6 o'clock a few of these patients will be meeting with me in room 242 to learn about what to expect before and after the operation. They will learn what they can do to speed recovery and remain as comfortable as possible. I think you'd enjoy meeting these patients and learning about your care. Would you like to join us?" If the patient is reluctant to join the group, exploration of his reason may result in his coming to the meeting.

When the group begins to assemble for the meeting, the nurse should introduce the patients to one another and allow a few minutes for them to become acquainted. At the beginning of the meeting the patients should be reminded of how long the meeting will last. This tends to motivate group members to accomplish their goals within that time. In addition, the nurse should summarize briefly what will be covered and explain how she expects the patients to participate. In the group organized for preoperative instruction, the nurse may suggest that the patients ask questions about each topic as it is being covered. She should also inform them that there will be 10 to 15 minutes at the end for other questions and informal discussion. Accuracy and confidence are increased when there is the two-way communication of discussion rather than the one-way communication inherent in the exclusive use of the lecture method.

The nurse may encourage participation during the meeting by making positive responses to each comment or question. Examples of positive responses are smiling, nodding in agreement, looking at the speaker, or making statements such as, "You're right about that," or "I'm glad you brought that up." Quiet members may be encouraged to participate if comments are directed at them. Or, they may be asked specific and easily answered questions such as, "Mr. Brown, you used IPPB during your last hospitalization. Would you tell the group what IPPB feels like?"

By observing the questions and comments of each group member the nurse may identify those patients who require further assistance. In any event, the patient should always have the opportunity to request or to engage in individual instruction in addition to attending the group. Sometimes a topic relevant to only one patient cannot be covered in the group, or a patient will have questions he did not wish to ask in front of the group. All members of the health team should be aware of the general content of the group meeting so that they can supplement this with patients on an individual basis.

Groups of parents or children. With only a few revisions the nurse may follow the previous suggestions in using the group situation to teach children about pain. The size of the group should remain small since children require more assistance in manipulating objects and understanding their purpose. The group should be kept small even if a parent accompanies each child. The nurse will then have to communicate on two different levels to reach both child and adult. Most of the topics appropriate to the adult group also need to be covered with a group of children. However, the method of teaching differs. The nurse relies less on verbal communication and provides more opportunities for the child to handle equipment and practice exercises. The children will learn through this type of play. The nurse can provide a central theme for the play by saying, "We are going to play hospital and find out what happens when a boy or girl goes to the hospital." She may use a doll to represent the patient and/or allow the children to select and alternate the roles of patient, nurse, parent and physician.

When the group is composed of parents only, the nurse may conduct the group in almost the same manner as she would if the parents were adult patients undergoing the painful event. More information might need to be included about visiting policies. Also, both lectures and discussion should include ways parents can help their children and how the parent feels when his child is ill and in pain.

Managing other people who come in contact with the patient. The people who come in contact with the patient in pain sometimes need as much help from the nurse as does the patient himself. These people include health team members such as nurses, physicians and physical therapists, loved ones such as husband or wife, parents, sweetheart, and friends or acquaintances. Each of these people may contribute something to the relief of the patient's pain, or at least they may avoid causing an increase in his pain. The nurse must identify in each of these people the potential for increasing or decreasing the patient's pain and interact with each person accordingly. The nurse's interactions with these people may include encouragement to continue effective actions, suggestions of ways they may assist the patient, and efforts to alleviate their anxieties or anger so that the patient's anxiety does not increase. When their anxieties or anger cannot be alleviated, the nurse may then alter the situation by removing that person from the patient's environment or by postponing a painful event when that is possible.

Any person, whether he is a friend or the physician, may assist with the patient's pain relief in almost any of the ways the nurse does. For example, a visitor may give accurate information about a painful experience similar to the patient's, make positive statements about the effectiveness of a pain relief measure the patient is employing, or provide an opportunity for the patient to discuss what his pain means to him. The visitor may also produce pain relief in ways not available to the nurse. A friend may provide hours of distraction, a loved one may help banish loneliness and anxiety, or a clergyman may assist the patient to mobilize spiritual resources. Because of the patient's respect for medical expertise, a physician's reassurance may be more valuable than the nurse's comments.

When a person contributes to the patient's pain relief, the nurse encourages him to continue. She may do this by mentioning to him what he has done and praising him for this action. For example, the nurse was present when the physician enthusiastically told Mrs. Ames that he was changing her medication to a new drug that should be even more effective in relieving her arthritic pain. Outside the room the nurse commented to the physician. "That was a great thing you did—telling Mrs. Ames how positive you were that this change in medication would help her pain. That kind of statement from a physician seems to help patients with pain." The physician smiled and said, "Yes, I guess it does." The nurse observed that on the following days this physician made similar positive statements to other patients, perhaps because the nurse had reinforced his behavior.

Comparable circumstances arise with people who are not members of the health team. For instance, as a result of an automobile accident Mr. Jackson was hospitalized with skeletal traction for a fractured femur. He was a bachelor without close relatives, and for a week he had no visitors. He occasionally commented that other patients were lucky to have company in the evenings. The nurse also noted that he always requested his oral analgesic during the evening visiting hours. One evening he was visited by a married couple whom he had seen socially about once a week prior to his accident. About 15 minutes after they arrived the wife walked outside the room and the nurse said to her, "I'm so glad you've come. Mr. Jackson needs visitors." The wife replied, "Are you sure? I was thinking we should leave. He looks like he would be in such pain." The nurse excused herself for a moment and went to look at Mr. Jackson. She found that he was engaged in a rather lively conversation and showed no signs of pain. The nurse returned to the wife and said, "He looks like he's having a good time. Did he say he was uncomfortable?" Further conversation with the wife revealed that Mr. Jackson had admitted some discomfort upon questioning, but had not referred to it again. The wife seemed frightened of the traction so the nurse explained its purpose and that it no longer caused severe pain. When the wife returned to the room she seemed relieved and the couple stayed until the end of visiting hours. Mr. Jackson did not request his analgesic during the visit. When the couple left the nurse encouraged them to return. She suggested that they could help the patient in another way by asking other friends to visit. For the rest of the week Mr. Jackson had visitors almost every night. He no longer requested his analgesic in the evenings, and he fell asleep easily after his visitors left. This illustrates how visitors provide a distraction that alleviates mild pain. This also demonstrates how the nurse can help visitors become aware of their beneficial influence, allay their anxieties about the patient's condition, and suggest additional ways of helping the patient.

Sometimes a family member who is very close to the patient such as a husband or parent is particularly concerned about ways to help the patient during painful experiences. Besides reinforcing whatever the family member is already doing to assist the patient, it may be necessary to make suggestions or help the family member figure out other means of assisting him. For example, based on her knowledge of the patient, the nurse may suggest to the relative a variety of ways to relieve the monotony that may contribute to pain. This need not involve the expenditure of money because the relative can bring from home books, photographs, a record player, a favorite food, games, or letters. For the child the parent may also bring a favorite toy or blanket. When it is indicated, the nurse may also suggest what the relative might say to the patient. She may encourage the relative to express his confidence in the medical management, point out signs of progress, or allow the patient to talk about the meaning of the painful experience. Sometimes a relative feels that he should be very jolly in front of the patient and avoid talking about topics that trouble the patient. When this does not seem to help the patient, the nurse may suggest to the relative that he encourage the patient to talk about whatever worries him. She may specify to the relative what may be causing the patient to worry, such as the implications of the cause of the pain or a fear of impending pain.

Another approach may be employed to involve the relative in assisting with the patient's pain relief. The nurse may ask the relative what he ordinarily does at home when the patient experiences some discomfort such as a backache or stomachache. This question may encourage the relative to utilize previously effective methods of assisting the patient with pain. This technique worked particularly well with Mr. Simons who was disturbed that his wife had developed a spinal headache following surgery. In addition to giving him some information about spinal headaches, the nurse asked if his wife had ever had headaches before and what he did about them. Mr. Simons replied that his wife occasionally had a severe migraine headache and that he usually brought her a lemon pie. He added, "That sounds so silly, but she loves it and it always makes her feel better. I guess I might as well try it now." Mrs. Simons was on a regular diet, so the pie was permissible. Within an hour Mrs. Simons was eating lemon pie. A wrinkled brow and muscle tension in her extremities were replaced with a smile and relaxation. Coincidentally, but appropriately, the remainder of the pie was kept on the unit in the refrigerator containing medications.

Handling sources of anxiety and anger in others. At times the patient's pain causes great anxiety and even anger in those who come in contact with him. These emotions may prevent a person from being able to assist the patient with pain relief. Or, these feelings may be conveyed to the patient, increasing his anxiety and decreasing his ability to cope with pain. It is especially unfortunate when anxiety or anger occurs in those people with the greatest potential for making significant contributions to the relief of the patient's pain. The people with this potential are most likely to be a loved one, the physician and the nurse. In this respect it is interesting to note that married persons seem to experience less pain than unmarried persons, perhaps because of the support given by the spouse (Bruegel). Unfortunately, the loved one, or the person with whom the patient has the closest affectional relationship, seems to be the most neglected resource for pain relief.

When anxiety or anger occurs in a person who could otherwise help the patient with pain relief, the nurse may manage the situation by first attempting to decrease the anxiety or anger. If this fails she may then remove the person from the patient's environment. Or, sometimes she can postpone the painful event until the person leaves voluntarily or controls his anger and anxiety. (Since anger and anxiety may occur in the reader as well as other people, the reader is reminded that the following comments may be helpful in handling these feelings in one's self.)

To assist people who demonstrate anger or anxiety in relation to the patient's pain experience, the nurse must understand and appreciate some of the possible causes of the anger or anxiety. One source of these feelings consists of those things that may also bother the patient. In other words, the threat or meaning of the pain may concern the patient and may also cause the physician, nurse or family member to be angry or anxious in the presence of the patient. For example, a physician severely reprimanded one patient for failing to report postoperative leg pain that had occurred the day before. Both physician and patient were concerned about the same thing—that the leg pain indicated a complication. The patient handled his anxiety by trying to deny the existence of the pain, and the physician coped with his own anxiety by becoming angry with the patient. Even if the threat or meaning of the patient's pain is not known to the patient, it may be a source of anxiety to others. A wife, for instance, may become tearful when her husband complains of pain because she fears it indicates a fatal illness. Both of these examples illustrate the fact that the threat or meaning of the patient's pain, whether or not it is shared by the patient, may cause anger or anxiety in those who come in contact with him.

A second source of anxiety or anger in those who come in contact with the patient is derived from frustrated attempts or desires to protect and help the patient. For example, when a patient adamantly refuses a pain relief measure suggested by the nurse, the nurse may feel ineffective and powerless. It is sometimes difficult for the nurse not to manifest anger. Her anger may be evident in her facial expression or the way she abruptly leaves the room. Another very common situation is the parent who miserably and anxiously stands by his child after an operation, unable to prevent the pain and knowing that the kiss that soothed so many hurts in the past may not work so well for this one.

In health team members there is a third source of anxiety and anger about the patient in pain. This arises from the desire to be professionally competent. For example, when the physician makes an unsuccessful attempt to perform a lumbar puncture, he may respond to the patient with anger or display anxiety. The physician's response may have little to do with his compassion for the patient's suffering. He may simply be reacting to a situation that threatens his competence.

When someone manifests anxiety or anger in the presence of the patient with pain, the nurse attempts to reduce these feelings. To do so she uses her knowledge of the possible causes of the anxiety or anger. Either during or following such a situation, the nurse may comment on or discuss some of the positive bases of the person's behavior. For example, Mr. Jones stayed with his three-year-old son Paul on the evening following Paul's open heart surgery. When the nurse helped Paul turn from side to side, Paul began to cry. Mr. Jones displayed his anxiety when he ordered his son in a harsh tone of voice, "Stop crying. You've got to do this." The nurse felt that the father's anxiety and seeming anger were more related to his concern for the child's condition than to the value he placed on stoic pain responses. Therefore, the nurse said to Mr. Jones, "It isn't easy to see your own child being hurt." Later, when Paul was sleeping, Mr. Jones left the room and the nurse followed him. She opened the conversation with Mr. Jones by saying, "It's so difficult for parents when their child is sick and they feel unable to help. Do you feel that way?" The father replied, "Oh, yes. I know he's getting along all right, but I worry anyway. All that coughing and turning. I guess it's necessary, but it hurts him. Seems like it might be pulling on something that could come loose." Mr. Jones was expressing his anxiety over the meaning of the pain. The nurse pursued this topic by encouraging him to talk about other concerns and by giving him appropriate information. Eventually Mr. Jones seemed to understand the purposes of the various painful procedures and was assured that the pain did not indicate a potential complication. The nurse then turned the conversation to the exploration of Mr. Jones' feelings of helplessness when his son was in pain. The nurse asked, "Is it hard for you to see Paul hurting?" Mr. Jones replied, "Yes it is. I don't know how to help him. If I could just do something." The nurse discovered that Mr. Jones ordinarily did not object if his child cried with pain. Therefore, she suggested that he allow Paul to cry now, adding that it might be very difficult for Paul to use his limited energy to try to keep from crying. The nurse also suggested other ways Mr. Jones could help Paul, such as holding his hand, helping him splint his incision when he moved, and moistening his lips with cool water. For the rest of the evening Mr. Jones followed these suggestions. He displayed no anger and very little anxiety in the presence of his son.

This example illustrates how the nurse may assist people who manifest anxiety and anger toward the patient in pain. The nurse helped Mr. Jones identify his feelings, provided information about the safety and purpose of the painful activities, and suggested ways Mr. Jones could assist his child. Most people, especially parents, respond eagerly to opportunities to discuss their fears and concerns related to the patient in pain.

A particularly important time to assist the parent with his anxiety related to the child is when the parent is informed in advance of his child's hospitalization. If the parent is highly anxious about what will happen, he may make no attempt to prepare the child for hospitalization. Later the child's anxiety about the strangeness of the hospital may contribute to his pain. Even worse than this is the example of the anxious child who is brought to the hospital when his parents have told him they are taking him shopping or to a movie. The nurse in the outpatient setting may be able to assist parents with their anxiety and help them to prepare the child for hospitalization. One way is to suggest that the parents and child tour the hospital a day or two prior to admission. Some hospitals conduct such tours on a regular basis. If the hospital does not do this, the parents can at least take the child to certain areas of the hospital where visitors are allowed. In this way both the parents and the child become familiar with the hospital in advance. On the day of admission, anxiety related to strange surroundings is not as great. The nurse in the outpatient setting may also wish to obtain literature that assists the parents to prepare their child for hospitalization.*

When a person manifests anxiety in the presence of the patient or expresses anger toward the patient during the pain experience, it may on occasion be necessary to remove that person from the patient's environment. This should be done only when the nurse has failed in her efforts to help the person control his feelings or when the nurse's other immediate responsibilities do not allow her the time to do so. For example, if Mr. Jones had been unable to benefit from his interaction with the nurse, it might have been necessary for the nurse to ask him to wait outside the room each time Paul had to turn or cough. Another situation in which a relative would probably have to be asked to leave is in an emergency, when the nurse does not have time to interact with the relative. If the angry or anxious person is significant to the patient, his potential ability to raise the patient's anxiety and thereby increase the perceived intensity of pain is as great as his potential for comfort. While the latter is what the nurse wishes to accomplish, realistically it is not always possible. Therefore, the angry and anxious person must sometimes be asked to leave the patient's room.

Even if a person is not especially anxious or angry, it may be advisable for him to be absent while a patient is experiencing pain, particularly severe pain. The nurse should observe the patient's response to pain when other people are present and discuss with the patient his preferences regarding the presence of others while he is in pain. Some patients prefer to be alone with their pain but may feel it is rude to ask others to leave. It is sometimes easier for the patient if the nurse assumes this task. In relation to the infant and toddler, it has been suggested that even the relatively calm parent be absent when a painful procedure is performed. This is contrary to the beliefs of some, but it is worth noting since it is often quite difficult to assist the very young

---

*Copies of a small booklet entitled "Your Child Goes to the Hospital" are available free of charge to the nurse or physician by writing to Ross Laboratories, 625 Cleveland Avenue, Columbus, Ohio 43216. This is an excellent little book written for parents. It assists the parents with many aspects of hospitalization, including preparing the young child for pain. The nurse may keep a copy in the waiting room and give a personal copy to parents when their child is scheduled for hospitalization.

child in pain. The reason given is that the young child who cannot understand explanations of procedures also cannot understand why his mother or father does not prevent the pain. If the parent is not present the child is spared the feeling that the parent is helping to hurt him (Webb). One opposing argument is based on the fact that the very young child often experiences anxiety over separation from his parent. If the child must cope with a painful experience, it seems senseless to impose an additional source of anxiety by separating him from his parent.

On occasion it is possible to postpone a painful event until the anxious or angry person has time to compose himself or until he has voluntarily ended his visit with the patient. For instance, if Mr. Jones had not benefited from his interaction with the nurse but had been visiting for only a brief period, the nurse could postpone turning for a few minutes until he left. Sometimes the physician becomes anxious in the presence of the patient and he, too, may benefit from the nurse's suggestion to postpone a painful procedure. For example, one physician made several unsuccessful attempts at a venipuncture on a child. He manifested his anxiety when he angrily told the child to stop crying and be still. The child cried even louder and became more active. At this point the nurse said, "It's almost impossible to do this on an active child. Shall we wait for him to calm down?" The physician nodded in agreement and returned an hour later, relaxed and confident.

Providing other sensory input. A common misconception about the treatment of the patient in pain is that he should be placed in a quiet environment and left undisturbed. The patient in pain is often subjected to a quiet room with dim lighting, no visitors or silent ones, and tiptoeing nurses. It is true that some patients prefer to be alone with their pain. And, for almost all patients in pain there is great value in rest and relaxation. However, very often, increasing stimulus input to the major sensory modalities can be an effective pain relief measure.

Two methods of increasing sensory input are (1) distraction and (2) touch or other forms of cutaneous stimulation. Distraction may involve any of the senses (smell and taste usually being less significant). Since distraction may include tactile stimuli, the reader may wonder why the use of cutaneous stimulation is singled out as a different method of increasing sensory input. The reason will be dealt with later in this section, but suffice it to say now that certain types of cutaneous stimulation do not act merely as distractions.

Distraction. A positive correlation exists between pain relief and distraction. Distraction may decrease perceived intensity of pain and/ or increase tolerance for pain. There are several explanations of the mechanism by which distraction contributes to pain relief. One of these is anxiety reduction. For a sensory stimulus to act as a distraction, the patient's attention must be focused on it and not on pain. Focusing of attention is well known as an effective maneuver for reducing anxiety. As we have already discussed, a decrease in anxiety contributes to pain relief.

Another reason that distraction results in pain relief is that distraction elicits responses that are incompatible with pain responses. Pain tends to draw attention to itself. Therefore, when the patient thinks about pain, he is making a pain response. However, when the patient focuses his attention on something else he is not making that particular pain response. The distraction itself may elicit other reactions, such as verbalization or physical activity, that are also incompatible with certain pain responses. The patient cannot talk about pain if he talks about something else, and he cannot rub an injured area with the same hand he uses to move a chess piece. This phenomenon is perhaps related to the resolution of cognitive dissonance. If a patient feels pain but acts as if he does not feel pain, he tends to be motivated to resolve this contradiction. One method of resolving the dissonance is to perceive a lesser intensity of pain or tolerate the pain for a longer period of time.

The principle of eliciting behaviors incompatible with pain responses is discussed at length in relation to distraction rather than some other pain relief measure. This is done only because the application of the principle is more easily observed when distraction is employed. Distraction itself requires that the patient make responses that are incompatible with pain. However, Sternbach (1968) points out that eliciting responses incompatible with pain is common to a variety of effective pain therapies; for example, hypnosis and relaxation techniques.

An especially interesting research study shows the pain relief value of distraction as compared to some other approaches to the patient in pain. In this research five groups of subjects were exposed to a painful stimulus. One group, the control group, received no instructions prior to the pain, and each of the remaining four groups received one of the following sets of instructions of what to do during the application of the stimulus: (1) to expect severe pain, (2) to describe out loud their momentary experiences, (3) to describe out loud a set of slides, and (4) to watch a clock and determine a tolerance goal for themselves. The greatest tolerance for pain was shown by the group describing the slides. In descending order of tolerance were those who watched the clock, those expecting severe pain, the group without instruction and the least tolerant were those describing the painful experience (Kanfer and Goldfoot). The two groups employing some form of distraction (describing the slides or watching the clock) were more tolerant of pain than the other groups. This also demonstrates that the more actively the patient participates in distraction the more effective the distraction is likely to be. Verbal description of the slides was more effective than clock-watching, probably because it required more active participation and therefore greater effort.

Distraction takes many forms, and obviously slides do not have to be used. To determine a possible and appropriate type of distraction for the patient the nurse should keep in mind that the effectiveness of distraction as a pain relief measure is usually enhanced (1) by maximizing, within reason, the patient's efforts or active participation such as having the patient talk out loud rather than silently think of something and (2) by involving two or more of the sensory modalities of vision, hearing, touch and movement such as having the patient look at pictures and outline them with his finger rather than simply looking at them.

Even if the form of distraction employed does not require the patient to look at anything, he should be cautioned to keep his eyes opened and focused on one object. For example, the woman in labor who is using the various breathing techniques of the Lamaze method should focus her eyes on an object, frequently referred to as a "concentration point." Or, the patient who is using his imagination as a form of distraction, such as remembering the details of a trip to the grocery store, should also focus his eyes on one point. Keeping the eyes open and focused prevents the tendency toward the less structured and more drifting form of thought that occurs with the eyes closed. Focusing on an object is also in itself a form of distraction from pain. In addition, focusing the eyes may make it slightly more difficult for the patient to engage in the major form of distraction such as imagining a trip or breathing rhythmically. Imposing this minor difficulty is desirable. The patient must then increase his efforts both to keep his eyes focused and to concentrate on or participate in the major form of distraction. It has been found that trying to ignore distracting stimuli while concentrating on a sensorimotor task is a particularly successful pain relief measure (Morgenstern).

Using distraction for pain relief. Distraction may be used for pain relief with patients of any age and pain of any intensity or duration if the distraction is properly chosen. Theoretically, distraction should provide at least some pain relief for any patient with any type of pain. The problem, of course, is that of finding a stimulus or set of stimuli that will distract the particular patient. Not all patients can be distracted by the same thing. Further, for intense pain the distractor must be unusually powerful to keep the patient's attention off the pain. And, if the pain is of long duration, the distractor or combination of distractors must be ones that the patient can continue to utilize in spite of mental and physical fatigue.

A few examples will illustrate the usage of distraction for pain of relatively brief duration but of varying intensities and in a wide range of ages. For a male infant being circumcised a pacifier or a bottle of milk may be used as a distractor. A four-year-old child receiving an injection can be asked to wiggle his toes, hold his mother's hand and look at her face. A ten-year-old child having a renal biopsy may be asked to count backwards or to sing a song and keep time by tapping his fingers. An adult having a painful dressing change may be asked to describe a series of pictures. A person having a myocardial infarction may be asked to imagine (gasping usually prevents much talking) walking down a familiar street. A nurse used this latter technique very effectively with one patient who had a myocardial infarction and had to wait 40 minutes for a physician to arrive and order an analgesic. This same technique as well as some of the others listed, may require the nurse's assistance. A brief suggestion or question from the nurse may help the patient keep talking or find a new topic to imagine. And, brief comments of praise such as "very good" may encourage the patient to continue the use of the distraction.

Usually, the longer the pain lasts, the greater variety of distractions is required. For example, the patient using the Lamaze method during the hours of labor has learned three different types of rhythmic breathing. These are slow chest breathing, panting, and panting and blowing. She employs them in that order, changing to the next breathing pattern when the current one is no longer effective in relieving discomfort. The need for some variation after a period of time is illustrated by one patient in labor who had progressed to the panting and blowing. She had been using this breathing pattern for about three hours. At that time and on her own initiative she varied the activity by adding a nodding of her head in rhythm with the breathing. This movement of the head is not taught in the Lamaze classes, but the patient's need for additional distraction prompted her to move her head. She later said that this addition not only helped but seemed to be essential.

An even greater variety of distractions is necessary for the patient with pain lasting months or even years. This type of pain may be experienced, for example, by the patient with arthritis. The nurse may need to assist the patient with long-lasting pain to structure his days so that he employs many types of distraction and changes from one to another after a short period of time. Many distractions cease to be distractions if they are utilized continuously for a long period. For example, watching television may become ineffective after three or four consecutive hours of viewing. Water coloring may become boring if it is done every day, month after month.

Sometimes a powerful distractor is not necessary for the effective relief of mild or moderate pain. It may be sufficient merely to prevent the occurrence of one of the types of sensory restriction that contribute to the patient's pain experience. In other words, providing a normal level and variety of meaningful sensory input may produce pain relief. For example, the patient with pain may be exposed to the perceptual monotony of lying in bed and staring at blank walls. He may experience pain relief if his environment is changed to one that contains a normal amount of stimuli such as visitors, television, games and pictures. Unless it is contraindicated, physical activity should be included to provide stimuli. The tactile kinesthetic input from physical exercise appears to reduce significantly the effects of sensory restriction of any kind (Schultz).

Distraction may be used either purposely or accidentally as a pain relief measure. Many people deliberately and almost naturally employ distraction when they experience pain. They may talk to themselves or others, mentally and silently solve mathematical puzzles, hum, or count acoustical tiles on the ceiling.

Other people benefit from distraction without consciously realizing what has happened. Sometimes neither the patient nor the nurse is aware that distraction is resulting in pain relief. This seemed evident in one patient's account of her painful experience. Mrs. Frank, hospitalized for thrombophlebitis, was relating to the day nurse an incident that had occurred the evening before. Around six o'clock that evening a plumber had come to fix a sudden and rather severe leak in the bathroom adjoining Mrs. Frank's room. Mrs. Frank cheerfully told the day nurse how she had turned on the light and talked with one of the evening nurses who stayed with her during the 15 minutes it took to repair the leak. The nurse on the day shift finally said to Mrs. Frank, "You seem to have enjoyed this. But why was the light out? Were you sleeping?" Mrs. Frank replied, "I wasn't sleeping. My legs ached, so I was just lying there, tossing and turning. The nurse had given me some pain pill around four o'clock but it didn't work. But she said I should turn out the light and try to rest. I guess when the leak occurred there wasn't much else she could do but let me turn on the light and talk to her." The day nurse then asked if Mrs. Frank's legs had bothered her while she was talking with the evening nurse. Mrs. Frank said, "No, now that I think of it. I did mention to her that I couldn't sleep because of the aching. When she left she said I should turn out the light and try again, but my legs bothered me again." The distraction of turning on the light and talking to someone was an effective pain relief measure for Mrs. Frank, but neither she nor the nurse appeared to realize this. Sleep is an important method of combating fatigue in the patient with pain, but Mrs. Frank was not relaxed or sleeping. It would have been more appropriate if the patient had been encouraged to use various methods of distraction. In fact, a powerful distractor did not seem necessary — the patient needed a normal amount of input to combat the effects of monotony. Later in the evening Mrs. Frank could have been given a sedative and/or a more potent analgesic to promote sleep.

Distraction is a potent method of pain relief, so much so that it may work even when the patient declares that he has no confidence in its effectiveness. For example, Mr. Tolbert had several painful dressing changes every day. The nurse suggested to him that during the dressing change he talk to her about baseball, a topic that interested him very much. Mr. Tolbert said, "I'll try it, but it won't work." He did try and it did not work. With the next dressing change the nurse said nothing about distraction. However, she began talking with Mr. Tolbert about a television program he had been watching. Mr. Tolbert did not grimace or say "ouch" as he had during the other dressing changes, and he participated actively in the discussion. Afterwards, the nurse pointed out to him that the distraction seemed to have provided some pain relief. Mr. Tolbert reluctantly agreed with this and said, "Maybe talking did work." When the nurse came into his room to do the next dressing change, Mr. Tolbert enthusiastically asked, "Well, what are we going to talk about this time?"

When the patient is experiencing severe pain or is very frightened about his pain, it is sometimes difficult to distract him. All of his attention may be focused on the sensation of pain and/or on the meaning of the pain. First the nurse must get his attention and then she must provide a novel stimulus. Two simple and effective ways of getting his attention are either to whisper in his ear or call him by his first name. The distracting stimulus initially should be a novel one that is quickly and simply stated, requiring a response from the patient. This type of approach was effective with Mrs. Jones. The patient was screaming with pain while the physician was doing a dressing change and manipulating drains. The nurse whispered to her, "Ruth, look at my face. What color are my eyes." The patient stopped screaming, looked at the nurse, and said, "Blue."

When the patient experiences pain relief from distraction without realizing it, he should be made aware of it and assisted to use other forms of distraction. The patient who is already consciously using distraction should be encouraged to continue its use, and the nurse should help him with other sources of distraction. This may include bringing books and magazines, introducing him to other patients, or being present during a painful event to help him keep talking about topics that distract him from pain. The following example illustrates these and many other important aspects of using distraction as a pain relief measure.

Mr. Wiley, 56 years old, was admitted with back pain. On the day of this interaction he was to have a myelogram to determine whether or not he had a ruptured disc. The nurse found that Mr. Wiley had had a myelogram several years before. His recollections of the sensations, duration and purpose of the procedure were accurate and rather complete. She then asked Mr. Wiley if he had ever used distraction as a means of relieving the almost constant discomfort in his back. Mr. Wiley replied that he had used several types of distraction very effectively. He said that when the discomfort in his back increased he often tried to watch television or initiate a conversation with his hospital roommate. The nurse decided that Mr. Wiley would be a good candidate for the use of distraction as a pain relief measure during the myelogram. There was the additional advantage that Mr. Wiley also had previously experienced a myelogram, and therefore there would be less tendency for the patient to focus on the procedure. A certain degree of familiarity could have been accomplished by rehearsal of the procedure if Mr. Wiley had not experienced it in the past. When a patient is not familiar with most of what is involved in a painful situation, it is difficult for him to abandon a natural tendency to try and protect himself from harm by attending to or watching what is happening. For instance, even an unexpected noise associated with the procedure may divert the patient's attention from the distraction to the painful event.

The nurse then said to Mr. Wiley, "You've told me that you found your last myelogram very uncomfortable. I don't think this one will bother you as much if you use distraction. But this may require a more powerful distraction than you have been using. Also, you may need to use more than one type of distraction. Would you like me to tell you what I have in mind?" In this statement the nurse did several important things. She avoided using the term pain, suggested the purposeful use of distraction, suggested that distraction was an effective pain relief measure, defined the limits of the distraction as a pain relief measure by implying that some discomfort would be felt, encouraged the patient to perform well by telling him that the effectiveness depended upon him, and involved the patient in a preliminary decision about the possibility of the distraction being effective.

When Mr. Wiley replied that he would like to hear the nurse's ideas, she proceeded to explain the use of describing pictures during the procedure. She said, "When the doctor begins the myelogram I will show you a series of pictures I've taken from several different magazines. You look at these pictures and talk to me about them, describing them in great detail. Pretend that you are competing for a prize given for the most detailed description of these pictures. Tell me everything you think about them—what is happening, colors, size, height, number of parts, or anything else that occurs to you. Keep talking all the time. When you seem to have described most of the picture I will show you another one. Would you like to see how this works with two pictures I have now?" Again, the nurse involved the patient in making a decision. After he consented, the nurse showed him the pictures and he described them. This rehearsal allowed the patient to become familiar with the type of distraction, but it did not provide enough practice for him to begin to find it easy and therefore less distracting. It also gave the nurse an opportunity to make suggestions about what to look for in the pictures, to caution the patient not to talk too fast or too slowly, and to identify any other problems the patient encountered.

The nurse praised Mr. Wiley for his performance and continued, "As you know, at times during the myelogram you will have to remain very still and quiet. You will have to cooperate with some directions from the doctor, x-ray technician or me. When those times occur, talking will not be allowed. Therefore, you will need another type of distraction. For this distraction I suggest that you decide now on something to imagine that is very pleasant. And, it should be interesting enough to command your attention. What can you think of that's especially pleasant and interesting to you?" Mr. Wiley thought for a few seconds and replied, "Sex with my wife." The nurse responded with, "That's an excellent idea. Don't think about it in the meantime or it may not be as interesting later on during the procedure."

Prior to the myelogram the nurse explained to the physician and the x-ray technician what the patient would be doing. She also asked them to use the word discomfort instead of pain, and she suggested that at times it might be best for her to relay their instructions to the patient since the patient would be focusing on her more than on them. Without the cooperation of others several things may occur that decrease the patient's ability to use distraction effectively. When the patient begins to describe the pictures, others may laugh or interrupt to obtain an explanation. Or, quite often the physician unnecessarily diverts the patient's attention from the distractor to the pain. Sometimes the nurse must caution the physician to avoid telling the patient about each step of the procedure, warning the patient that he may feel pain, or asking the patient if he does feel pain. The occurrence of these difficulties may be controlled by adequate explanation to others prior to the procedure and by reminders during the procedure.

Throughout the myelogram Mr. Wiley used distraction but not in exactly the form that had been planned. He began by describing the pictures, but after about two minutes the nurse noted that he was beginning to use the pictures to remind him of personal experiences. He began talking about these experiences instead of describing the pictures. Gradually he no longer looked at the pictures, but he looked at the nurse and talked continuously about various topics that interested him. The nurse occasionally praised him with "excellent" or "very good." She did not attempt to get him to describe the pictures again because talking about other topics seemed to be an effective distraction in that Mr. Wiley did not manifest signs of discomfort. In addition, the nurse recalled that conversation was a method of distraction Mr. Wiley had used in the past. Frequently a patient either reverts to a distraction he has used previously or he refuses from the beginning to try another type of distraction. This is understandable in terms of the theory of operant conditioning. If a type of distraction has been used successfully in the past, pain relief has rewarded its usage and increased the likelihood that it will be used in the future.

Mr. Wiley's myelogram was unusually long and difficult, but he wrinkled his forehead and squinted his eyes only about four times. Once his body jerked rather violently when the needle hit a spinal nerve. There were no other manifestations of pain. After the myelogram the nurse asked Mr. Wiley to evaluate the usefulness of the distractions of talking and imagining. He described them as "very effective" and said that this myelogram "was not nearly as bad as the last one." The nurse asked specifically whether or not he had imagined sexual activity with his wife. He replied affirmatively, remarking again that it was effective. Mr. Wiley later commented about the procedure, "I knew it hurt but I didn't care." This is a particularly interesting statement since, as we shall see later, this is precisely the effect that morphine has on pain.

Lamaze method (*PPM*). The Lamaze or psycho-prophylactic method (PPM) of preparation for childbirth achieves pain relief through other means besides the use of distraction. Nevertheless, a portion of the method will be described briefly here because (1) the rhythmic breathing patterns and the eye focus can be used effectively as distractors for patients other than those in labor and (2) the nurse should be able to assist the patient who uses the Lamaze method during labor.*

The following explanation does not prepare the nurse for teaching the Lamaze method to expectant mothers. Teachers accredited by the American Society for Psycho-Prophylaxis in Obstetrics are available for that purpose. However, with sufficient study, practice and experience, the nurse may teach some aspects of the Lamaze method to laboring patients who have not been exposed to it.

The three rhythmic breathing patterns of the Lamaze method are:
1. Slow chest breathing. Inhalation through the nose and exhalation

---

*More complete information about the Lamaze method may be obtained in the paperback book *Six Practical Lessons for an Easier Childbirth* by Elisabeth Bing (1969).

through the lips, taking six to nine breaths per minute. The patient may maintain a constant rhythm by counting silently and slowly "in, 1, 2, out, 1, 2, 3, 4." This is used during the preliminary period of labor until it is no longer an effective pain relief measure.

2. Panting. Inhalation and exhalation through the mouth. Panting is shallow and begins slowly, accelerating as the contraction increases and decelerating as it subsides. The patient maintains a 4/4 rhythm by silently singing a 4/4 song such as "Yankee Doodle" or by counting silently to four, emphasizing the count of one. This is used during the more active stage of labor when contractions are about three minutes apart.

3. Panting and blowing. The patient pants in the same manner as above but pants four, six or eight times and then blows, accelerating and decelerating the rate of panting according to the intensity of the contraction. Again, the patient may count silently to maintain the four, six or eight count rhythm she has chosen. This is used during transition.

Each of the breathing patterns is practiced daily for several weeks prior to labor, but during labor they are used only with the contractions and not between contractions. Each breathing pattern is accompanied by a deep breath at the beginning and at the end of the contraction. Also, during each contraction the patient's eyes are open and focused on a "concentration point," usually a preselected object brought from home such as a mobile or a sea shell. With the first two breathing patterns, slow chest breathing and panting, abdominal massage is utilized. The patient or someone else such as her husband uses both hands and massages upward from the pubic area and then outward and down from the fundus. The patient is taught to remain completely relaxed physically at all times, both during and between contractions. If at all possible, the patient should not be disturbed during a contraction, and efforts should be made not to obstruct her view of the "concentration point." If the patient ceases to use the breathing patterns during a contraction and begins to complain of discomfort, the the most helpful measure usually is for the nurse (or husband) to have the patient look at her and breathe as she is breathing. Or, the nurse may count the rhythm out loud for the patient. This means the nurse must know which breathing pattern the patient is using, and in some cases the nurse must also be able to breathe in that way.

Hyperventilation may occur in some patients during the usage of panting or panting and blowing. This does not occur often with patients who have practiced the breathing patterns for several weeks prior to labor. Initial symptoms of hyperventilation are visual difficulties, dizziness or tingling around the lips. The patient is taught to recognize these symptoms and to breathe into a paper bag when they occur.

For many brief episodes of pain other than labor contractions, a patient may be taught one of the breathing patterns and use a "concentration point" to achieve pain relief. This works well during the time interval between administration and absorption of an analgesic or postoperatively when ambulation or turning is painful. Another example occurred with Miss Bell, who was hospitalized for a severe vaginal infection. She was allowed to inject her own vaginal medication, ordered every three hours. She described an intense burning pain starting 30 seconds after injection of the medication and lasting about one minute. The nurse taught this patient to use rhythmic panting during this time, and the patient said this effectively relieved the pain.

Cutaneous stimulation. The remainder of this section on providing other sensory input for the patient in pain will be devoted to the use of touch or cutaneous stimulation. Some types of touch may serve as distractors. For example, when the patient is in pain, the cool touch of the nurse's hand or a moist cloth on the forehead may provide a sensation other than pain on which the patient may focus. Other types of touch such as a backrub may enhance general relaxation. Cutaneous stimulation in the form of moist heat may relax painfully contracted muscles. The cutaneous stimulation of an ice pack may numb a painful area or reduce swelling. Having the child squeeze his ear lobes with the thumb and index finger of each hand, a very effective method of pain relief for intramuscular injections, provides both distraction and cutaneous stimulation. Touch in the form of holding the patient's hand is often used to reduce anxiety and meet the dependency needs that may result from pain. Frequently, a person in pain may be observed to apply his own cutaneous stimulation such as pressing his finger nails into the palms of his hands or rubbing or holding the painful area. Hence, several types of touch or cutaneous stimulation may contribute to pain relief in a variety of ways.

Is there some physiological mechanism that accounts for the fact that cutaneous stimulation of various types is a universal and common method of pain relief? One answer is provided by the gate control theory mentioned in Chapter 3. According to this theory, pain relief may be achieved by selectively enhancing the large fiber input. Cutaneous fibers are large-diameter afferent fibers. Therefore, the transmission of pain impulses (carried by small-diameter fibers) from the spinal cord to the brain may be inhibited by cutaneous stimulation. This mechanism has been used to explain why certain types of cutaneous stimulation relieve pain in the following conditions. Causalgia has been relieved by bathing the limb in gently moving water followed by massage. In one case, pain of central nervous system origin was controlled when the patient tapped his fingers on a hard surface. In general, vibration reduces low intensity pain (but it increases high intensity pain). Some amputees obtain relief from phantom limb pain by tapping the stump gently with a rubber mallet (but heavier pressure aggravates the pain). Electroanalgesia, which stimulates free nerve endings in the skin, effectively relieves chronic intractable pain in some persons ("Pain"; Melzack and Wall, 1965).

Another explanation for the pain relief achieved by cutaneous stimulation is the notion of extinction or perceptual dominance. As mentioned in Chapter 3, intense pain in one area of the body raises the threshold for milder pain in another area. Intense pain also raises the threshold for other sensory inputs such as auditory stimuli. It is possible that this relationship may be reversed so that sensory input other than pain may extinguish pain or raise its threshold. For example, the intensity of deep pains may be reduced by applying non-noxious tactile pressure or heat to the skin. To be effective, the intensity of the non-noxious cutaneous stimulation must be just below the intensity that would produce discomfort. The resulting pain relief is felt to be related to the general phenomenon of extinction, or the elevation of perception threshold for one sensory stimulus while another is being applied (Wolff and Wolf).

Extinction would seem to be a likely explanation for the effects of audio analgesia. The use of intense auditory stimulation (i.e., music) to suppress the pain of dental drilling was very popular with dentists in the 1960's. Eventually audio analgesia was abandoned because it did not work with all patients. Research indicates that extinction is not the mechanism responsible for effective pain relief with audio analgesia. The auditory input does not actually produce analgesia, but it may increase tolerance for pain. When this effect occurs, it appears to be due to the patient's active use of the auditory input as a distraction. Increased pain tolerance occurs more frequently when the auditory stimulation is intense *and* when it is preceded by a strong suggestion that it abolishes pain (Melzack, Weisz and Sprague). Therefore, auditory stimuli do not appear to contribute to pain relief by elevating the threshold for pain or by decreasing pain impulses.

However, touch or cutaneous stimulation often contribute to pain relief by abolishing or decreasing the pain impulses. This effect may be explained by the gate control theory or by the phenomenon of extinction. With each patient the nurse probably will need to experiment on a trial-and-error basis to determine which area or areas of the body should be stimulated and which type of stimulation is required. The large cutaneous afferent fibers may be stimulated by massage, pressure, vibration, bathing, or the application of menthol rubbing agents. Sometimes intense stimulation will not be as effective as moderate stimulation. Regarding the area to be stimulated, the nurse may try the skin directly over an internal pain, the skin surrounding an external injury, or the area on the opposite side of the body corresponding to the painful site. In general, sensory inputs of moderate or high intensity applied to widespread areas of the body should effectively inhibit the transmission of pain impulses to the brain and thereby decrease or abolish pain (Melzack, 1970 b).

Two patients illustrate the effective usage of cutaneous stimulation for pain relief. The first patient, Mrs. Flynn, was in skeletal traction for the treatment of a fractured femur. Her most frequent complaint was of pain in her knee. The nurse tried a moderate intensity of massage to the knee for about 45 seconds. Mrs. Flynn reported that the pain was relieved for an hour afterwards. However, more intense massage did not relieve the pain. This supports the previously mentioned point that moderate intensity of cutaneous stimulation is often more effective than high intensity.

The second patient, Mr. Matthews, had a below-knee amputation, performed seven days previously because of severe arterosclerosis. Mr. Matthews described his pain as "barking" in his stump, and he requested his narcotic analgesic every three hours. Cutaneous stimulation was used for the first time when Mr. Matthews complained of the "barking" but was not allowed to have his analgesic for another hour. The nurse suggested and explained cutaneous stimulation to Mr. Matthews by saying, "Let's put some pressure above your knee. This should interrupt the pain messages to the brain." Mr. Matthews was anxious to try this. The nurse applied mild to moderate pressure to the anterior surface of his leg. This did not provide pain relief, but Mr. Matthews suggested that the pressure be applied all around his leg since the pain circumscribed his stump. Pressure was applied in this manner for about one minute, and it effectively relieved Mr. Matthews' pain for one hour.

The effectiveness of the abdominal massage used along with other aspects of the Lamaze method during labor may be due to tactile inputs superceding pain impulses. It is interesting to note that the abdominal massage is used only with the first two types of breathing patterns. The third and last breathing pattern, panting and blowing, is employed during transition. Possibly the more intense discomfort that may accompany transition does not respond to the rather moderate cutaneous stimulation of abdominal massage.

Promoting rest and relaxation. General relaxation of the skeletal muscles and sufficient rest and sleep contribute to pain relief but in a more subtle fashion than many of the other pain-relief measures. In Chapter 3 we noted that physical strain, which may be caused by spasm or contraction of skeletal muscles, may be a source of noxious stimuli. Tense skeletal muscles may also contribute to fatigue. Fatigue leaves the patient with less energy to cope with pain, and it also may produce a state of arousal in which the patient is prone to indulge in horrid fantasies about his pain. Muscle tension and fatigue not only contribute to the pain experience but are themselves often a result of pain. In some patients a vicious cycle may be initiated. Pain causes muscle tension and fatigue and these two symptoms in turn increase the subjective experience of pain. It is important to combat this occurrence by promoting rest and relaxation.

Sleep. Adequate sleep is one way to provide rest and relaxation. To determine what the patient needs to sleep the nurse must assess carefully whether or not the patient is sleeping or has slept. In addition, she should ask the patient to evaluate the type of sleep he is experiencing under conditions of discomfort. Many times the nurse's notes read "a good night" or "slept well." But, the next morning the patient is restless, tense and complains that he hardly slept at all or that he slept poorly. Often it is assumed that the patient is sleeping if his eyes are closed and he is relatively motionless when in fact he is merely trying to relax or go to sleep. Or, the patient may actually be sleeping; but if he evaluates his sleep as poor, the nurse should realize that he needs assistance. Research has identified many objective differences between what a person subjectively calls a good sleep and a poor sleep. For example, the person who says he sleeps poorly takes longer to fall asleep, is more restless, and dreams less than the person who says he sleeps well (*Current Research on Sleep and Dreams*).

In addition to employing a variety of pain relief measures while the patient is awake, several other nursing activities may promote restful and effective sleep. Medication is helpful for some patients. If the patient is sufficiently tired and is experiencing only a mild intensity of pain, he may be able to sleep unaided. But some patients may require a sedative. Others, especially those in severe pain, may be unable to sleep unless they receive both an analgesic and a sedative. Very often an analgesic is necessary since the patient is usually fatigued when it is time to sleep. This fatigue and the need to relax in a quiet environment may preclude the use of other pain relief measures such as distraction. If the analgesic relieves most of the pain and assists the patient to relax, this medication may be all that is necessary to promote sleep. On the other hand, the patient may require a sedative in addition to the analgesic. In general, the sedative alone should not be relied upon to relieve pain that is keeping the patient awake. Alcoholic beverages, muscle relaxants, or tranquilizers are sometimes substituted for sedatives. Again, depending upon the type of pain, muscle relaxants and tranquilizers do not necessarily relieve pain. However, they may enhance the effectiveness of an analgesic administered simultaneously.

A reasonably quiet environment is usually an aid to sleep. It is not always the level of sound that disturbs sleep, but the fact that the patient is not accustomed to the sounds. Almost everyone has experienced the difficulty of sleeping in a strange place with unfamiliar background noises. Hospitals can be very noisy places and much of the noise cannot be prevented. But if the nurse pays attention to this noise factor she may be able to eliminate some of the sounds. Explaining to the patient the sources of some noises may assist him to ignore them even in his sleep. Or, the patient may sleep better if he turns on a radio station programming music, since this may block out other sounds. If the patient, such as a postoperative patient, must be awakened periodically for various procedures, the nurse should try to minimize the number of disturbances. She may time the procedures so that as many as possible are performed during one period of wakefulness. It is probably also wise to avoid, when possible, awakening the patient during REM (rapid eye movement) sleep. A certain amount of REM sleep appears to be an important aspect of a "good" sleep (*Current Research on Sleep and Dreams*).

Many of the suggested approaches to pain relief also apply to the promotion of sleep. For example, the nurse may explore with the patient why he cannot sleep and what usually helps him to do so. Positive statements about the effectiveness of sleep-promoting measures may also be helpful.

Relaxation. Relaxation may contribute to sleep because it tends to abolish both mental and physical tension. But there is another reason for promoting relaxation in the patient with pain: it is itself a form of pain relief. Relaxation may decrease the amount of noxious stimuli in a variety of conditions. For example, relaxation of the abdominal muscles decreases the amount of discomfort associated with abdominal incisions or uterine contractions. Certain Eastern philosophies suggest the value of a relaxed response to pain, maintaining that the willingness to yield to pain and react naturally often makes further reactions unnecessary (Watts). Related to this is the fact that generalized relaxation of the skeletal muscles is one of several responses that is incompatible with pain responses. The production of these responses is an important aspect of many pain relief measures (see discussion of this under the section on providing other sensory input). Relaxation is an integral part of such pain therapies as the Lamaze and Read methods of childbirth and the hypnotic induction and trance.

A particularly interesting research study adds another dimension to the value of relaxation in pain relief. This study hypothesized that an individual's evaluation of the intensity of pain is in part a function of his evaluation of his own overt behavioral response to pain. In testing this, they found that when a person was allowed to withdraw from a painful stimulus he evaluated the stimulus as more painful than he did when he suppressed the avoidance response (Bandler, Madaras and Bem). To some extent it appears that on a subconscious level the patient says to himself, "This must be painful because I am so tense (or, because I am trying to escape)." This indicates that encouraging a person to relax instead of maintaining muscle tension or making escape responses will assist the patient to perceive a decreased intensity of pain.

In some cases relaxation may not decrease the perceived intensity of pain, as the above study suggests, but it may increase the tolerance for pain. An interesting clinical observation is that some patients receiving medication for pain, especially those receiving pentobarbital, report no change or slight change in the intensity of pain. However, they do not want further medication. They appear to be quite comfortable and free of tension (Beecher, 1956 c). In other words, when they are relaxed they do not appear to be bothered by the pain.

There are at least three ways to promote relaxation and thereby contribute to pain relief. First, general comfort measures assist the patient to relax. Proper positioning, smooth sheets, comfortable bed clothes, adequate ventilation and acceptable room temperature are but a few of the many measures the nurse may employ. Of particular importance is the back rub that so many patients find comforting and relaxing. General comfort measures should not be overlooked, but they will not be discussed in detail here, since they are covered in basic textbooks.

A second method of promoting relaxation is through the use of muscle relaxants or certain tranquilizers that also have some muscle relaxant properties. Muscle relaxants are frequently given in the treatment of painful muscle spasm. They are also valuable when only muscle tension is present or when muscle spasm is less obvious such as the reflexive muscle spasm following surgical incision. The use of medication to provide relaxation that contributes to pain relief is illustrated by Miss Brown, who had an infected wound on her leg. Dressing changes were done three times a day, and she responded to these with complaints of pain and with constant tension in the muscles of her neck and extremities. She described the pain as a "twitching" in the wound. Forty-five minutes prior to the next dressing change she received 10 mg. of Valium, a tranquilizer with some muscle relaxant properties. She responded to the dressing change with only periodic muscle tension, and she stated that the pain was considerably less. Valium seems to have contributed to pain relief by replacing tension with relaxation and by reducing the reflexive muscle spasms in the wound.

The third method of achieving relaxation is by teaching or training the patient to relax. Both the Maternity Center Association* and the

*see *Psychophysical Preparation for Childbearing: Guidelines for Teaching,* 1965

Lamaze methods of childbirth demonstrate that this can be done. Patients are trained in advance to respond to the discomfort of labor with relaxation instead of muscle tension. In both methods relaxation is a significant aspect of achieving a comfortable labor and delivery. But, in neither method is there agreement on how relaxation contributes to pain relief. Perhaps relaxation contributes to pain relief because it sometimes decreases noxious stimuli during a contraction, or because it is a response incompatible with pain responses. In addition to these reasons, two other explanations have been advanced. These are based on the idea that relaxation is used differently by different people. The first explanation suggests that relaxation produces a state of increased suggestibility in some persons. In this state, explicit and implicit suggestions of comfort are received favorably. The increased suggestibility may be due to the occurrence of a mild hypnotic state or to the establishment of a psychotherapeutic relationship. In either case, the relaxed person seems to be very susceptible to what is said and done. The second explanation suggests that other persons use relaxation in a rather mechanical way. These patients concentrate on maintaining relaxation. This type of relaxation focuses attention, a form of distraction that may in turn contribute to pain relief (Chertok).

There are a number of ways to teach the patient to relax in response to pain. We will begin by discussing the methods used in the Maternity Center Association and the Lamaze classes, both quite similar, which have been successful and are based on many years of experience. Knowing how this relaxation is taught will enable the nurse to assist the patient in labor who is using either of these methods. The nurse also will be able to teach other types of patients how to relax.

At least several weeks prior to delivery, relaxation is practiced daily. The mother assumes a comfortable and well supported position, usually lying down with her knees and hips slightly flexed. She takes a deep breath, contracts one or two extremities such as one arm or one arm and one leg, and relaxes the remainder of her body. During this exercise someone must check the extremities and other areas of the body such as the neck to determine whether or not they are in the proper state of relaxation or contraction. Through this exercise the mother learns to control relaxation of her body. The exercise is not used during labor; it is preparation for relaxing during labor and delivery. Relaxing the rest of the body while one area is contracted is difficult; the natural tendency is for the whole body to become tense. By learning to relax while an arm, for example, is contracted, the mother is better able to achieve total relaxation later during a uterine contraction.

In most cases a signal is established as a command to relax. The signal is used during labor to assist the mother to relax. For example, if the mother's legs become tense during a contraction the established signal is used to call her attention to the tension and to the need to relax. The signal may be tapping the legs or the words "relax your legs."

There is one signal that seems to be quite useful in assisting with relaxation in a variety of patients in addition to the labor patient. It is the instruction, "Breathe in, relax as you breathe out." This signal is useful with most patients, especially those who have not been trained in relaxation, because a big sigh is often associated with relaxation. In many people sighing and relaxing have been paired often enough in the past for sighing to have conditioned the response of relaxation. The signal to relax at the end of a big breath takes advantage of the conditioned response of relaxation. This is probably one of the reasons why both the Lamaze and the Maternity Center Association methods of childbirth teach the patient to take a deep breath at the beginning of each contraction. The signal of breathing and relaxing is not ordinarily used during a contraction because the patient may be concentrating on a breathing pattern, but it may be used if she becomes excessively tense.

The instruction to take a deep breath and relax may be employed to promote relaxation in patients with a variety of conditions. It may be used with both children and adults. If possible the patient should practice breathing and relaxing two or three times prior to a painful experience. But the instruction is simple enough that practice is not essential unless the patient is a young child. For example, Jim, a six year old, was cooperative during injections. He remained very still, but his body was generally tense and his gluteal muscles were contracted. Between injections the nurse taught Jim to "take a deep breath, let go of the air, and go limp as a rag doll." He practiced this while he was lying on his stomach. His toes pointed toward the midline to further gluteal muscle relaxation. Jim thought this was fun and seemed to view it as a game. The nurse praised him for being able to relax and explained that the next time he had an injection she would ask him to do this. For the next injection Jim assumed the correct position and followed the nurse's instructions regarding breathing and relaxing. Generalized tension was absent and the gluteal muscles were relaxed. Afterwards Jim said, "That was lots better than the others."

When a patient is being instructed preoperatively in the various postoperative exercises, the notion of relaxing with the deep breathing can be included. If the patient is to have an upper abdominal incision or thoracic surgery, deep breathing probably will be uncomfortable although it is necessary. However, the nurse can modify that aspect of the breathing that is to accompany relaxation. She may suggest that after the exercises he take several slow breaths that are not deep enough to be uncomfortable. He can try to relax completely at each exhalation. Even without practice any adult patient who has pain that is not affected by deep breathing may be instructed to breathe in deeply and relax as he breathes out.

Some patients may need more assistance with general relaxation of the body than that provided by the simple breathing and relaxing measure. This measure may not result in sufficient relaxation for an especially tense patient. For example, Miss Hardy was admitted to the hospital with a "whiplash" injury with possible involvement of the cervical disk. She benefited from both the breathing-relaxing technique and the application of the practiced relaxation used in the childbirth methods. The painful muscle spasms in her neck and shoulders increased her tendency toward generalized muscle tension. This tendency results from any type of pain but it is increased when muscles in one area of the body, such as the neck in this case, are in a state of contraction that is not under voluntary control. Miss Hardy's generalized muscle tension resulted from her neck pain. This tension seemed to contribute to increased contraction of muscles in the neck and shoulders, increasing the pain. It was important to interrupt the cycle of pain and muscle tension; therefore, relaxation techniques were used along with other pain relief measures. The nurse explained to Miss Hardy that relaxation would help her be less bothered by the discomfort and that the relaxation might also decrease the severity of the muscle spasms in her neck and shoulders. The nurse instructed the patient to breathe in and relax her whole body as she breathed out. This resulted in some decrease in general muscle tension. However, when the nurse attempted to move the patient's extremities she found that they were not limp and did not move freely. The nurse then said, "When I pick up your arm or leg it should be limp and should fall back on the bed when I release it. You can see that you are still tense enough that I can't freely move this arm, and it remains suspended when I let go. Try to relax this arm completely." The nurse continued to move the arm until the patient achieved complete relaxation in the arm. This was accompanied by greater relaxation in the other extremities, and the nurse pointed this out to Miss Hardy. Throughout the day the nurse returned every hour or so to practice the relaxation for a few minutes with the patient. After about five hours the patient seemed to have mastered it. Miss Hardy said she employed it when the neck and shoulder pain increased and that it effectively decreased the pain. She also stated that when she concentrated on relaxing, the pain did not bother her as much. These comments indicate that the relaxation techniques probably decreased the intensity of the noxious stimuli and increased her tolerance for the remaining pain.

Clearly, relaxation techniques may assist a variety of patients with pain. However, as is true with many other pain relief measures, relaxation will not be viewed by all patients as a valuable aid to coping with pain. As we noted in Chapter 3, for example, the Irishman may consciously use relaxation to deal with pain. But the Italian may reject its usage since his method of handling pain is to remain as active as possible.

Using behavior therapy. In this book many references have been made to the ways in which operant and classical conditioning are related to the patient's behavioral responses to pain. In Chapter 3 we mentioned how operant conditioning is involved in the transmission of cultural expectations regarding appropriate pain responses. We also discussed how classical conditioning accounts for some of the effects of personal past experiences with pain. Behavior therapy is one of several terms used to denote a form of treatment or teaching-learning process that employs the principles of classical and operant conditioning. Behavior therapy is used mostly in the fields of mental illness and retardation, but its use is by no means restricted to these areas. In fact, most of us apply the principles daily without realizing it. Every time we praise someone's behavior we are employing the principle of operant conditioning. According to this principle a behavior will tend to occur more frequently if it is consistently followed by reward such as praise. When a mother tries to quiet a crying infant by holding him, she is relying to some extent upon the principle of classical conditioning. That is, a response (freedom from tension) to a stimulus (being fed) can be put under the control of a different stimulus (being held) by having the two stimuli occur together often enough (holding the baby and feeding him day after day).

Some types of behavior therapy are particularly appropriate to the management of the patient in pain. In this chapter there are repeated suggestions that the nurse reward the patient in some way such as praising him when he learns to relax or to use a distraction. This is a very simple and easy application of operant conditioning. Reward increases the likelihood that the patient will continue to make these responses to pain. The greatest reward for making these responses is, of course, pain relief. If the patient experiences pain relief almost every time he employs a certain pain relief measure, he will tend to use it more frequently. However, until the patient learns how to use some pain relief measures such as relaxation, he may not be reinforced or rewarded by pain relief. Therefore, until pain relief occurs, it is helpful if the nurse offers reinforcements in the form of attention or verbal praise.

Reinforcement or reward may also be useful in preventing further pain. Sometimes the patient must subject himself to painful activity such as postoperative ambulation in order to prevent a more painful condition such as thrombophlebitis. Verbal praise for the adult or a piece of candy for the child may encourage efforts to cooperate. Another usage of reinforcement to decrease the duration of pain and prevent further pain is illustrated by Clay, five years old, who was having a lumbar puncture. The procedure was in progress when the nurse entered the room. Clay was crying loudly and making many body movements to escape. The nurse knew that his activity might result in more than one puncture attempt and that his crying would prolong the procedure by making it difficult to obtain a pressure reading. Hence, the nurse decided to attempt the use of reinforcement. Each time Clay stopped crying long enough to take a breath the nurse said, "Clay, you're being so quiet now. That's very good." She continued to make statements like this as long as he was quiet. She said nothing when he was crying. In this way the nurse rewarded cessation of crying; she did not reward crying—she simply ignored it. Frequently a child gets more attention for crying than for being quiet during a procedure, but in this case the nurse did not allow that to happen. Clay's periods of being quiet began to increase in frequency and duration. The nurse then began the same reinforcement process for his activity. Within about three minutes Clay was quiet and inactive often enough for the procedure to be completed without delay.

At this point it is important to clarify what this author considers appropriate usage of giving and withholding reinforcement of responses to pain. Withholding reinforcement of pain responses should be done only when the pain response itself will prolong or increase pain. This is illustrated in Clay's case discussed above. In other circumstances pain responses should be reinforced in the form of conveying acceptance and respect for the patient's manner of responding to pain. In her efforts to obtain a change in behavioral response that indicates pain relief, the nurse should rely upon the pain relief measure. She should not employ withholding of reinforcement to elicit this behavior change. For example, if the patient cries in response to pain, the nurse may hope for a cessation of crying as an indication of pain relief. She should rely upon the pain relief measure to achieve cessation of crying. She should not attempt to cause cessation of crying by ignoring the patient when he cries.

Classical conditioning as well as operant conditioning may be employed to obtain pain relief. This possibility was demonstrated many years ago in one of Pavlov's (1928) classical conditioning experiments with dogs. Some dogs repeatedly received food immediately after being painfully shocked, burned or cut. They eventually responded to the pain stimuli as signals for food. Instead of making pain responses such as howling, they would salivate in response to the noxious stimuli.

The Lamaze method of childbirth, which originated in Russia and was based on the Pavlovian theory, relies to some extent upon conditioning. Both operant and classical conditioning appear to be involved. One explanation of this conditioning process is as follows. With training and practice the mother acquires a set of conditioned reflexes with which to respond to labor. These replace unconditioned, reflexive responses such as muscle tension. Hence, the mother responds to contractions with the conditioned responses of relaxation and a rhythmic breathing pattern. The mother learns this prior to labor. She begins by learning the responses of relaxation and the breathing patterns in response to specific verbal stimuli. She then learns to relax and use a certain breathing pattern in response to a contraction. The principle of classical conditioning comes into play when relaxing and rhythmic breathing are brought under the control of another stimulus—the contraction—instead of the verbal command. Since this is taught before labor, the stimulus of the contraction must be simulated in the form of the words "contraction begins" and the physical stimulus of someone squeezing an area of the body. In other words, once the mother has learned the behavior of rhythmic breathing in response to verbal instruction, she then learns to respond with this behavior when a contraction is simulated. The husband may say, "Contraction begins." At the same time he simulates a contraction by placing his hand on her arm and squeezing with gradually increasing intensity up to a point and then gradually decreasing intensity. The principle of operant conditioning is also inherent in this learning process since the mother is praised both subtly and obviously as she learns these responses and since there is the implied reward of future pain relief.

The type of conditioning process used in the Lamaze method may also be employed with patients who will be experiencing other types of discomfort. For instance, preoperatively a patient may be taught relaxation and a rhythmic breathing pattern. The responses of relaxation and the breathing pattern may then be paired with the stimulus of discomfort in the operative site. This may be simulated by the nurse applying pressure and pulling the skin in the operative area, having the patient simultaneously respond with relaxation and the breathing pattern. Or, certain types of distraction may be substituted for the responses of relaxation and rhythmic breathing. Using this conditioning process, the patient may be taught to respond to pain with responses that are incompatible with pain responses, thereby achieving a measure of pain relief.

Desensitization. Some other types of behavior therapy may contribute to pain relief if they are used to decrease the patient's fear and anxiety about a painful experience. Patients who are particularly frightened of pain or pain-related stimuli may benefit from a form of desensitization (Layton). In preparation for using this, the nurse determines those things that frighten the patient. She then constructs a hierarchy arranged in order from those stimuli that are the most frightening to those that are the least frightening. Next she provides an environment that is pleasurable and free of anxiety-producing stimuli. Such an environment may simply consist of helping the patient become relaxed and comfortable in bed, perhaps through the use of a back rub. The nurse begins the process of desensitization by talking with the patient about those things that are the least frightening. She continues up the hierarchy until the patient shows some signs of fear. She stops at this point and dwells on those things that do not elicit anxiety, trying again later to discuss the more frightening items. Eventually the patient may become desensitized to at least some of those things that are rather frightening to him. Whether or not this form of desensitization is employed in a strict sense, the nurse should nevertheless remember that in general it is well not to persist in discussing or familiarizing a patient with things that elicit excessive anxiety. This should be a more gradual process.

The notion of introducing potentially anxiety-producing stimuli when the patient is experiencing pleasure and the idea of introducing frightening stimuli gradually can easily be applied to the child. For example, if a child is admitted to the hospital, new people and equipment may be introduced during periods when he is free of other stressors. If a child is responding with pleasure or comfort to some situation when the unfamiliar is introduced, he is more likely to associate the unfamiliar with a comfortable situation. The nurse might begin by playing with the child and giving him a lollipop. If he is having a good time, she might suggest that he take his lollipop and go for a walk with her. If he is to have surgery, she could take him to the recovery room and show him some people in operating room attire, a blood pressure cuff, oxygen tent and any number of other things he will be seeing again later, before or after surgery. If at any point the child becomes upset, the nurse should stop. For instance, if he becomes frightened of touching the leads on a cardioscope, the nurse may take him away, play with him, and return him to the cardioscope later.

If the child responds with anxiety when an object is introduced for a second or third time, another form of desensitization may be used. This is often called "fading in" and is especially applicable to children (Whitney, 1966 b). Again, it entails giving the child something very pleasurable to do, but this time the frightening object is very gradually brought closer to him. For example, if ice cream is a big treat for him, he can be taken to his room and given some ice cream to eat. While he is eating, the cardioscope can gradually be brought closer to him. At first the cardioscope might have to be 15 or 20 feet away from him outside his door. It could be brought closer by a few feet every minute or so. If at any point the child becomes frightened, the cardioscope can be put back a few feet. In this way his fear of the equipment is slowly decreased.

Shaping. Another technique that can be employed in the same situation is "shaping," a type of operant conditioning (Whitney, 1966 a). This involves reinforcing successive approximations toward a desired response, and it reflects the principle of teaching the simple before the complex. In the above situation, for example, the cardioscope could be put far enough away from the child that he feels safe. Each time he looked at the monitor he could be praised, given candy, or some other type of reward. After he had done this for a while, then he would be rewarded only if he took a step toward the monitor. In this way he is rewarded for slowly overcoming fear of the cardioscope and getting closer and closer to it. He is allowed to set his own pace for overcoming his fear. And, the use of a reward may increase his feelings of accomplishment and make him aware that others are proud of him.

Administering pharmacological agents. Analgesics are usually defined as drugs that relieve pain without loss of consciousness. According to this loose definition the majority of medications could at times with certain patients be classified as analgesics. For example, penicillin is not ordinarily thought of as an analgesic, but if its administration cures a painful wound infection, penicillin could be called an analgesic by this definition. However, the term is usually reserved for those drugs that relieve pain without having potent curative powers. Meperidine, for instance, relieves the pain of a wound infection without curing the infection. Broadly there are two classes of analgesics: (1) nonspecific ones such as morphine and aspirin that relieve a variety of types of pain, and (2) specific ones such as Pyridium, a urinary tract analgesic, that relieve only a certain type of pain.

This section on administering pharmacological agents focuses on some of the nursing activities that may enhance the pain relief potential of both analgesics and other medications such as antibiotics that may contribute to pain relief in certain patients. No attempt will be made to cover all the important aspects of these medications, such as dosages, contraindications, etc.; for these the nurse is referred to a pharmacology book. We will begin by taking a quick look at what the commercial drug market reveals about the general public's attitude toward pain medication.

Public attitudes about medication. In the United States many industries spend a tremendous amount of money advertising various pain-relieving products. Whether this originally represented a response to the public's need or the creation of that need in the public, the fact remains that a large number of people in the United States seek pain relief through medication. The advertised, non-prescription products are used mostly in the self-treatment of self-diagnosed conditions. But all of this establishes in the minds of many people an association between pain relief and medication. Consequently, when a person becomes a patient he may continue to expect some pain relief to come in the form of a medication. In support of this, interviews with surgical patients revealed that they expected the nurse to respond to their complaints of pain by giving a medication (McBride, 1967). Therefore, with regard to the use of pain-relieving drugs, the nurse should realize that many patients may have had little if any experience with other pain relief methods. Further, patients do not necessarily view the nurse as possessing the ability to offer a variety of pain relief measures.

The fact that some patients rely upon medication for the relief of many types of pain and do not expect much more from the nurse than medication has several implications for nursing care. Often the nurse will need to educate the patient to the fact that she can assist with pain relief in ways other than medication. If the patient is reluctant to employ other pain relief measures, the nurse probably will have to introduce these measures together with medication. (Of course, this use of other pain relief measures in addition to analgesics is a sound method of achieving the greatest degree of pain relief for many patients.) Further, even if the patient claims that he receives pain relief from measures such as distraction or relaxation, he may continue to be reluctant to use them and may insist upon relying solely on medication. However, the nurse should not allow this state of affairs to cause her to resort to the automatic administration of a medication for pain relief. She should continue to assess the situation carefully and in addition to medication should offer any measures the patient may accept such as a back rub or repositioning. And she should always continue to employ the types of approaches suggested in the sections on establishing a relationship with the patient and teaching the patient about pain. The importance of these interactions with the patient is indicated by the findings of one study in which some patients received analgesics without the nurse's exploring the meaning of the pain. Fifty percent of these patients experienced no pain relief (McBride, 1967).

Nonanalgesics. Many patients who experience pain benefit from understanding how nonanalgesics contribute to pain relief. Numerous drugs are used for the purpose of curing or controlling the cause of the pain. Therefore, they are given on a regular schedule, not on a p.r.n. basis for episodes of pain. Pain relief is not their main purpose but is an indication that they are effectively accomplishing their purpose. These types of drugs may include antibiotics given for painful infections, vasodilators and anticoagulants that control the painful effects of decreased circulation in peripheral vascular diseases, diuretics that decrease the discomfort of edema,and antispasmodics for the treatment of hypermotility of the gastrointestinal tract.

Some patients with pain will be primarily concerned with obtaining a cure for the cause of the pain. They may not easily accept drugs that are merely palliative. Other patients may have an opposite point of view, being more concerned with immediate pain relief by whatever means are available. With either type of patient it is important to explain how nonanalgesic medications contribute to pain relief. However, the nurse's approach will differ according to which method the patient values. For example, Mr. Newman was admitted for treatment of a painfully infected injury to his left leg. When the nurse entered to administer his first injection of an antibiotic, he said, "That's not any kind of dope, is it?" After the nurse explained that it was an antibiotic and not a narcotic, Mr. Newman continued, "When will that do some good?" Through further exploration the nurse ascertained that he was asking when his wound would improve. The nurse explained that the physician believed the antibiotic would result in some improvement within a few days. Mr. Newman responded, "Then the pain ought to be less in a few days?" The nurse replied, "Yes, but do you want some other medicine for pain in the meantime?" Mr. Newman refused this offer by saying, "I'll just wait a few days and let these shots (antibiotics) take care of it. I don't want any dope." Knowing that efforts were being made to cure the cause of the pain seemed to increase Mr. Newman's tolerance for pain. Although the nurse explained that he could ask the physician for aspirin or some other non-narcotic drugs, Mr. Newman refused. He seemed satisfied with the eventual pain relief from the antibiotic. This interaction revealed that Mr. Newman valued a cure for the cause of the pain. Therefore, each time the nurse administered one of his medications, such as antibiotic injections, oral vitamins and antibiotic ointments to the wound, she explained how it contributed to curing the infection.

In a similar situation, also involving an infected wound, the patient, Miss Sawyer, voiced a different attitude toward drugs and pain relief. While the nurse was making the bed, Miss Sawyer commented, "The doctor says my operation is infected and he's going to start giving me some shots. I hope they start soon. It really hurts." This suggested that Miss Sawyer was more concerned with immediate pain relief than with a cure for the cause of the pain. This was confirmed a few minutes later when Miss Sawyer said, "I don't care what's causing it (the pain). I just want it to go away." In addition to discussing other pain relief measures the nurse explained, "These shots are antibiotics that will help control the infection. The infection is causing the discomfort you started feeling yesterday. In a way these shots will make you feel better because they will help clear up the infection that causes the discomfort. Of course, it will take a few days before these particular shots have a noticeable effect on the infection. But there are other things that will help in the meantime." Although this explanation includes information about the curative aspect, it stresses the pain-relieving contribution of the antibiotics because the patient was more concerned with pain relief than a cure for the cause of the pain.

Specific analgesics. The specific analgesics that relieve only a certain type of pain include ergotamine for migraine or vascular headaches, colchicine for gout pain, Pyridium for urinary tract discomfort, and Nitroglycerine for angina pectoris. Patients who receive analgesics that are specific for a particular type of pain need to understand two things: (1) the medication should not (and often cannot) be used to relieve other types of pain and (2) usually the drug replaces the need for nonspecific analgesics. This should prevent confusion, illustrated by the following episode. During the postpartum period Mrs. Beck developed burning on urination and asked for her p.r.n. dosage of codeine orally. The nurse administered the codeine without asking what type of pain Mrs. Beck was experiencing. When the physician arrived Mrs. Beck reported her symptoms and an order for Pyridium 100 mg. orally p.r.n. was written. The next time Mrs. Beck experienced the burning, she requested "my new pill and the white pain pill." Discussion revealed that Mrs. Beck thought both medications were necessary for relief of the burning. The nurse explained that the Pyridium would relieve the burning much more effectively than the codeine alone. She also suggested that the Pyridium alone probably was all that was necessary to relieve the burning. Since Mrs. Beck was experiencing no other type of discomfort, Pyridium was the only medication given. Mrs. Beck reported later that it effectively relieved the burning pain.

Nonspecific analgesics. In administering nonspecific analgesics, which have an ability to relieve pain of various types, the nurse has perhaps a wider range of responsibilities than with the administration of most other groups of medications. Because these analgesics are most often prescribed on a p.r.n. basis, the nurse must be able to determine whether or not and when they should be given. With other drugs this decision usually is made by the physician. Also, because the nurse and not the physician ordinarily has the greatest amount of contact with the patient receiving analgesics, she must be able to evaluate the effectiveness of the drug in relieving the particular patient's pain. With many other types of drugs such as antibiotics or anticoagulants, the physician evaluates their effectiveness after several doses through laboratory tests and other physical signs. But, the nurse must evaluate the result of an analgesic after each administration. Also, when more than one analgesic is prescribed, the nurse must be able to choose the more appropriate one. Further, to a large extent the physician relies upon the nurse's decisions and observations when he prescribes or changes the administration of an analgesic. The nurse's contribution to the physician's plan of treatment is enhanced if she understands some of the alternatives in the administration of analgesics, such as routes of administration, dosages, and combinations of drugs.

Guidelines for carrying out some of these responsibilities are discussed in other parts of this book. Chapters 2 and 6 on assessment and evaluation assist the nurse in determining the effectiveness of an analgesic in relieving a particular patient's pain. Chapter 3 mentions some significant factors that enable the nurse to determine the need or desirability of an analgesic, but a few additional comments will be made in this section. Also included in the following discussion is some general information about selection of analgesics and alternatives in their administration.

Certain types of patients will tend to rely on analgesics more than other pain-relief measures. Several factors influence the patient's desire for an analgesic. Often it is not so much the severity of the patient's pain, but his willingness or ability to tolerate the pain and/or to use other methods of pain relief. For example, the patient may utilize various methods such as relaxation and positioning, but to obtain the maximum degree of pain relief he may also request an analgesic. Or, in some situations, postoperatively for example, the patient will require an analgesic because his level of arousal and fatigue prevents him from employing those measures that require his active participation, such as distraction. Another type of patient will prefer to remain passive during pain experiences either because this is his nature or because illness and pain provide him with a socially acceptable opportunity to be more dependent. Such a patient may accept measures that allow him to continue his passivity, such as back rubs and discussion of the meaning of pain. Often, however, he also desires an analgesic. Another patient will not want to endure any pain, no matter how mild, if it can be alleviated. Typical of such a patient is the comment, "My headache isn't really bad, but why bother with it if some aspirin will get rid of it?" At the opposite extreme, of course, is the patient who is reluctant to take any kind of drug and would rather experience pain than risk the potential dangers or side effects of medication.

There are some situations in which it is advisable for the nurse to assume the initiative in giving an analgesic rather than to wait for the patient to request it. As a rule, all pain-relief measures are more effective if they are used before pain occurs or before it becomes severe. Therefore, if the patient requires an analgesic among other things for pain relief, he should be cautioned to request it early in the pain experience. In addition, the nurse should be alert to impending pain. This is especially true if a time is approaching when the patient will be able to sleep uninterrupted if he does not awaken with pain. For example, it was eleven o'clock one evening when the nurse finished assisting Mrs. Layton to ambulate and void for the first time following delivery. Upon questioning, Mrs. Layton said that she was not experiencing much discomfort from the episiotomy and felt she would be able to sleep. The nurse pointed out to the patient that sensation was beginning to return since the spinal anesthetic was given ten hours previously. She added that Mrs. Layton might awaken with more discomfort in a few hours. To assure a better sleep and to prevent the discomfort from becoming severe, the nurse persuaded the patient to take her analgesic then. As a result the patient reported the next morning that she slept well for eight hours.

In the care of children with pain another circumstance may arise in which the nurse must sometimes assume the responsibility for the decision that a p.r.n. analgesic be given. Some children do not like oral medications, and many try to avoid injections at all costs. Consequently, a child may deny pain upon questioning or say that he does not need anything for his pain. In this case the nurse must assess the presence and severity of pain by observing other behaviors. If pain seems to be present, the nurse may feel it is advisable to administer an analgesic in spite of the child's protests. This is an especially important action for the nurse to take if the child's pain is interfering with his recovery, such as preventing rest and sleep or making it difficult for him to cooperate with coughing postoperatively.

In working with the physician to choose an effective analgesic for the patient the nurse needs to understand some of the facts related to the potency of analgesics. As a general principle, the potency of the analgesic selected to alleviate pain should be based on the patient behavior that indicates the severity of the pain and *not* on the degree of pathology involved. For instance, if the patient reports mild pain following extensive surgery, he will require a less potent analgesic for pain relief than will the patient who reports severe pain following the same or less extensive surgery. On the basis of the patient's evaluation of the intensity of his pain the nurse may need to request the physician to increase or decrease the potency of the analgesic.

Parenteral analgesics. Usually the most potent analgesics are parenteral narcotics. Morphine was isolated over 150 years ago, and despite continued research, no analgesic has been found that offers greater pain relief with fewer side effects. Other narcotic analgesics differ in speed and duration of action and in cost. However, when they are administered in dosages that provide a degree of analgesia comparable to morphine, the undesirable side effects are also comparable (Masson). There are, of course, individual differences in drug tolerance. Occasionally a patient will have fewer side effects from one drug than another. However, this discussion will focus mainly on morphine, and most of the comments will apply to the parenteral administration of other narcotic analgesics such as meperidine.

One of the most interesting aspects of morphine is the way in which it causes pain relief. Most of the time morphine does not appreciably alter the source of noxious stimuli, and sometimes it does not decrease the perception of pain. As incredible as it may seem, one study found that after the administration of morphine the individuals actually improved in their ability to perceive differences in the intensities of painful stimuli (Hill, *et al.*). The predominant pain relief action of morphine appears to be associated with the production of euphoria that decreases anxiety, alters the reaction to pain and increases the tolerance for it. This is illustrated by Mr. Cook who was admitted to the emergency room with multiple lacerations received in a fall. He received 10 mg. of morphine subcutaneously, and 30 minutes later he was asked to evaluate the amount of discomfort he was experiencing. He commented, "The pain is still there. In a way it hurts just as much as before, but I feel fine now. It doesn't bother me any more." Obviously the morphine did not decrease the noxious stimuli or even decrease the perceived intensity of the pain. But, morphine did appear to relieve Mr. Cook's anxiety and increase his tolerance for pain. Sometimes this reduction in anxiety will also result in a decrease in the perceived intensity of pain. As a result the patient will report that the pain is less severe and that it bothers him less. In a few circumstances, morphine will alter somewhat the noxious stimuli. In the patient with myocardial infarction, for example, the decrease in anxiety contributes to a decrease in the heart's need for oxygen and thereby decreases the painful stimuli of ischemia in the cardiac muscles.

Because morphine and other narcotic analgesics do not always decrease the perceived intensity of pain, the nurse should be careful not to suggest to the patient that the pain sensation will disappear after such analgesics are given. After receiving morphine or meperidine many patients have commented that they expected their pain to "go away." They were perplexed and somewhat upset that this did not happen. Therefore, the nurse should accompany the administration of morphine with more realistic statements such as "This will help you relax and feel more comfortable," or "This will keep the discomfort from bothering you so much."

Since morphine most consistently contributes to pain relief by reducing anxiety and creating a feeling of euphoria, it is frequently and effectively employed during the anticipation of pain. Anxiety may be quite high during the anticipatory phase of pain. Giving morphine at this time provides greater pain relief than administering the drug after the onset of pain. The idea that pain should be present before a narcotic is administered is not true. When the patient is anxious about an impending painful event that will require a narcotic analgesic, the medication should be administered before the pain occurs. Mrs. Dobbs illustrates this type of situation. In the afternoon of her second day following hemorrhoidectomy Mrs. Dobbs announced that she felt a strong urge to have a bowel movement and that she dreaded the pain.

The nurse immediately gave the patient's p.r.n. dose of morphine subcutaneously. Morphine decreased the patient's anxiety and 30 minutes later the patient had a bowel movement. By giving the analgesic during the anticipation of pain, the nurse achieved greater and more complete pain relief than if she had administered the analgesic during or after the bowel movement. In this case of giving morphine in the anticipation phase of pain, there was also the advantage of preventing Mrs. Dobbs from delaying the bowel movement because of fear of pain.

Morphine is far more potent when it is given parenterally than when it is given orally. Also, the potency can be adjusted to some extent by varying the dosage. For example, if the patient receives adequate relief from severe pain with 10 mg. of morphine subcutaneously, 5 mg. probably will relieve moderate pain. On the other hand, if the patient does not receive sufficient pain relief with 10 mg., increasing the dosage to 15 mg. may only prolong the duration of pain relief. It may cause only a slight increase in pain relief but a considerable increase in side effects. Therefore, if a sizeable increase in dosage does not significantly increase pain relief, there is little to be gained by a further increase in dosage. If greater pain relief is desired without increasing the dosage, the physician may administer morphine intravenously. Only 1 to 2 mg. intravenously at intervals of 10 to 30 minutes may result in greater pain relief with a smaller total dosage. This intravenous method is particularly effective with pain that occurs the first few hours postoperatively (Masson).

This knowledge of the potency of parenteral narcotics and of the possibilities for increasing and decreasing the potency should assist the nurse in making suggestions regarding the analgesic for the particular patient. It will also help her select the appropriate analgesic when more than one has been prescribed. For example, Mr. Maupin was receiving meperidine 50 mg. intramuscularly and tolerating it well with no side effects. However, the dosage did not sufficiently relieve his postoperative pain. Rather than changing to a comparatively larger dosage of another narcotic, such as 10 mg. of morphine, the nurse suggested increasing the dosage of meperidine from 50 mg. to 100 mg. Meperidine 100 mg. is considered to be equal to 10 mg. of morphine, but continuing with the same drug that Mr. Maupin was tolerating well minimized the possibility of side effects. In another situation the nurse had to choose between meperidine 50 mg. orally and the same drug and dosage intramuscularly. Both were ordered on a p.r.n. basis. The patient, Miss Reynolds, suffered a variety of discomforts in several locations due to metastasis of a malignancy. On this occasion the patient complained of mild discomfort in her right lower chest, one of the areas of metastasis. Among other pain relief measures, the nurse suggested the oral analgesic which Miss Reynolds agreed should alleviate the pain. Had the pain been severe, the nurse would have suggested the more potent analgesic which was the same dosage administered intramuscularly.

Although narcotic analgesics are more potent when they are administered parenterally, increased potency is not the only reason for parenteral administration. Psychological or physiological stressors tend to decrease absorption in the gastrointestinal tract, contraindicating the use of oral analgesics. For example, if the patient is highly anxious, regardless of the cause, absorption of an oral analgesic may be delayed. Or, absorption of drugs may be decreased considerably following any type of surgical procedure. This is particularly true if the gastrointestinal tract is the site of surgery or if certain anesthetics such as ether have been administered. When these types of stresses occur, oral analgesics may be much less effective and usually should not be employed until normal function of the gastrointestinal tract resumes.

Oral analgesics. When absorption from the gastrointestinal tract is adequate and when pain is mild or, in some cases, moderate, oral analgesics are indicated. They cause less discomfort than parenteral medications, and they eliminate the possibility of infection from an injection. The potency of oral analgesics may be increased somewhat by administering them when the patient's stomach is empty. For example, if the patient requests an oral analgesic at the time lunch is served, the nurse may suggest that he delay lunch for 30 minutes after taking the medication. In this way a larger amount will be absorbed more rapidly.

There are probably more types of oral analgesics than parenteral ones. Surprisingly enough, ordinary aspirin is one of the most effective. Some oral narcotics are more effective than aspirin, but studies have shown that oral administration of 60 mg. of codeine, a very common oral narcotic, or 10 mg. of morphine orally is no more effective than 0.6 Gm. of aspirin orally (Keats). Parenterally codeine is more effective than aspirin, but it is not as effective as morphine parenterally. The potency of aspirin tends to be underestimated by both health team members and patients perhaps because it is available without a prescription. For this reason alone, many adult patients may obtain more pain relief from another drug. As we have mentioned before, regardless of the pain relief measure employed, the patient's and the nurse's belief about its effectiveness will influence the amount of pain relief achieved.

In addition to its potency, aspirin has the advantage of not possessing the side effects or addiction potential of oral narcotics. Studies indicate that the average adult may take dosages of 0.3 to 0.6 Gm. of aspirin several times a day over a period of days without harm. In fact, an adult may take 20 to 50 tablets a day for several years before signs of chronic poisoning appear. Of course, aspirin does have side effects and is contraindicated in some conditions. There are on record a few instances of abuse in which a person has taken huge amounts of aspirin daily for many years (Boyd). Nevertheless, when an oral analgesic is indicated, aspirin should be considered because oral narcotics more easily produce undesirable side effects such as respiratory depression and constipation, not to mention addiction. For pain in infants and young children, aspirin is usually sufficiently safe and potent to provide adequate pain relief. Narcotics are rarely used in this age group. If aspirin cannot be taken orally it is often given rectally.

Originally the mechanism by which aspirin relieves pain was felt to be similar to that of narcotics. It was thought that aspirin altered the patient's reaction to the pain without decreasing the perception of the pain. However, recent research indicates that aspirin acts peripherally. Apparently it decreases the amount of painful stimuli by blocking the generation of impulses at the chemoreceptors for pain (Lim). Whereas morphine promotes pain relief by enabling the patient to tolerate the pain, aspirin decreases the perception of pain by decreasing the actual amount of painful stimuli transmitted. Therefore, the nurse can expect that when the patient obtains pain relief from aspirin he will tend to report a decrease in the intensity of pain. He probably will not say that his pain is the same but no longer bothers him. If the patient does make a statement similar to the latter the nurse may consider the possibility that the fact of receiving a medication lowered his anxiety. This patient might benefit from other measures that decrease anxiety.

Alcohol. Another oral substance that is not usually considered an analgesic but does in fact have analgesic properties is ethyl alcohol. Alcohol acts as a tranquilizer, reducing anxiety that may be increasing the pain. More related to its analgesic power, though, is the tendency for it to produce a "reducer," one of the algesic types mentioned in Chapter 3. This means that alcohol causes the person to underestimate what he perceives. Everyone knows it is dangerous to drive an automobile after consuming alcoholic beverages because judgment is poor. The driver underestimates such things as the amount of time it will take him to stop the car, the speed at which he is driving, and the distance between himself and other objects. This underestimation of sensory input also applies to pain. Hence, after ingesting alcohol the patient with pain will tend to underestimate the intensity of pain (Sternbach, 1968).

The nurse may have many opportunities, with the physician's permission, to encourage the patient to use small amounts of alcohol for pain relief. Some hospitals serve alcohol at the patient's request, or the physician may prescribe it during hospitalization. In outpatient settings the nurse may encounter a patient who is not opposed to alcoholic beverages and whose condition permits their use. If he has pain the nurse may suggest that he employ alcohol in addition to other pain relief measures.

Alcohol as well as many drugs may be abused by the patient, and the nurse should be alert to this. To prevent abuse, the nurse may stress small amounts of alcohol and the use of beer or wine rather than distilled spirits. When the same concentration of alcohol is consumed by drinking beer, wine, or distilled spirits, the blood-alcohol level is lower for beer or wine. The nurse may also suggest that the alcoholic beverage be taken with meals since this further lowers the blood-alcohol level (*Uses of Wine in Medical Practice*).

Tranquilizers, antidepressants and sedatives. Besides analgesics, other types of drugs may be employed to promote pain relief. The most common ones are tranquilizers, antidepressants and sedatives. One of these may be given instead of or in addition to analgesics. They may be prescribed on a regular schedule or on a p.r.n. basis. They are used mainly to decrease the anxiety or depression contributing to the patient's pain. To this extent they are similar to narcotic analgesics in that they modify the patient's reaction to pain. But, with the possible exception of the amphetamines, these drugs do not produce the euphoria of narcotic analgesics such as morphine. Therefore, they are not usually as effective as narcotic analgesics. Often they are administered for the purpose of reducing the frequency and/or dosage of analgesics. This is of particular importance in patients with long-term pain or in patients who develop undesirable side effects from narcotic analgesics. For example, one patient achieved adequate pain relief from meperidine 75 mg. intramuscularly, but he also experienced the side effects of nausea and vomiting. The nurse suggested to the physician a lower dosage of meperidine combined with a tranquilizer that had an antiemetic effect. The physician prescribed meperidine 40 mg. and chlorpromazine 25 mg. intramuscularly to be given at the same time. The patient obtained comparable pain relief without nausea and vomiting.

The patient with pain of long duration is understandably prone to develop anxiety or depression over his condition. In addition to other efforts to decrease or control these feelings, tranquilizers or antidepressants may be indicated. For instance, one patient who was hospitalized for many weeks for a series of skin grafts to burned areas of her body was requesting analgesics an average of four or five times a day. She manifested considerable anxiety over her physical appearance and the weeks of painful events. The nurse consulted with the physician regarding this anxiety and the frequent need for analgesics. The physician prescribed Valium, a tranquilizer, three times a day. As a result the patient reduced her request for analgesics to once or twice a day. Apparently the tranquilizer decreased the anxiety and thereby contributed to some pain relief.

The patient with pain who suspects or knows that he has a fatal illness presents a difficult and complicated situation. He may or may not be able to work through his feelings about death. The depression or grief and mourning that may occur at some point in his illness has various relationships to his pain. Very often this depression either increases the perceived intensity of pain or is handled by focusing on the pain. Being unable to ask for and receive the promise of a cure, he may express his feelings of helplessness and hopelessness and his desire for something to be done by talking about his pain and by making frequent requests for pain relief. When depression rather than anxiety is associated with pain, pain relief may be enhanced through the use of antidepressants such as Elavil and Tofranil. However, these drugs should never be used as a substitute for assisting the patient to discuss his feelings to the extent he is able.

Sedatives were discussed in the section on promoting rest and relaxation. However, it is worth reminding the reader that although sedatives alone may relieve minor discomforts they are rarely effective with severe pain.

Addiction. A discussion of pharmacological agents that provide pain relief would be incomplete without a few remarks about addiction. The term "addiction" usually refers to the development of both psychological and physiological dependence upon a drug after prolonged use. This is coupled with a need to increase the dosage to maintain a particular therapeutic effect. For example, a person addicted to morphine would crave the psychological effect of euphoria. In addition he would require a certain dosage of morphine for the maintenance of ordinary cellular activities. And he would need increasingly larger doses to achieve the same degree of pain relief originally obtained with a smaller dosage.

With regard to the addiction of the patient in pain, the most likely offender is the parenterally administered narcotic analgesic. The dosage is usually higher and the euphoria greater than is the case with oral narcotics. Addiction is sometimes the reason given for withholding a narcotic that is desperately needed by the patient for pain relief. Therefore, the nurse should have a realistic understanding of when addiction may and may not be a problem. When addiction exists it is a serious problem. However, it is not likely to occur if narcotic injections are given for severe pain over a period of days. Not only is this a relatively short period of time, but the reinforcement the patient receives after administration of the narcotic is pain relief. The reinforcement that ordinarily contributes to addiction is not pain relief; it is the euphoria associated with the reduction of drives the person does not seem able to gratify. It is obvious that the majority of addicts are not taking narcotics to relieve a localized sensation of pain. The evidence suggests that they are taking narcotics to reduce anxiety and drives such as hunger and sex. Other people satisfy these drives and feelings in a variety of ways, but the addict can achieve a sense of well-being only by injecting a narcotic. When a patient in pain desires only the reward of pain relief from a narcotic, he is not likely to want the narcotic when his pain subsides. In addition to this, it has been suggested that the passive recipient of a narcotic, such as the hospitalized patient, is not as prone to addiction. When the recipient of a narcotic is passive, he has less control over the reinforcement, whether it is drive reduction or pain reduction. He does not give the injection to himself whenever he desires it; this is controlled by others. Therefore, he is less likely to become addicted than someone who posesses a narcotic and can determine when or if he gives himself an injection (Nichols).

The possibility of addiction may be considered in the following situations: when a patient receives narcotics regularly for a period of two to four weeks (Rayport); when the patient is more interested in the experience of well-being than in pain relief; or when increasing dosages of narcotics are necessary to relieve the same intensity of pain. If the nurse suspects addiction, she should consult the physician and explain her reasons for being concerned. She should not take the responsibility of withholding narcotics.

The following situation illustrates how the nurse's knowledge of the characteristics of addiction enabled her to assume a calm and reasonable attitude toward assisting a patient. Mrs. Henderson was admitted to the hospital for the treatment of various external and internal injuries sustained in an automobile accident. On the first day of hospitalization she was placed in skeletal traction for a fractured femur. On the third day a splenectomy was performed. By the fifth day all internal bleeding had ceased and the external lacerations were healing without complication. At the beginning of hospitalization the physician prescribed 75 mg. of meperidine intramuscularly p.r.n. every three to four hours. Mrs. Henderson requested this three to four times a day until the sixth day when she requested it only twice. On the morning of the seventh day she had received one injection of meperidine when the physician said to her, "You're getting along very well now. It looks like you'll recover smoothly from here on. I don't believe you'll need these pain shots any more. I'm switching you to a pill of the same drug with a lower dosage, and in a few days aspirin ought to be all you'll need." Mrs. Henderson replied immediately and with a note of panic, "Oh no! Please don't take away my pain shots. I can't stand it. The pain can be so bad." At the end of these pleas there were tears in her eyes. The physician replied, "Well, I'll have to think about it. You've been on those shots a long time. I'll see. I'll be back later."

Later the nurse talked with the physician. He explained that he was inclined to discontinue the injections because he feared addiction, adding that Mrs. Henderson's emotional response to his suggestion only increased his apprehension. The nurse had cared for Mrs. Henderson for several days. She drew upon her observations of the patient and her understanding of addiction to make the following comments and suggestions. She reminded the physician that the possibility of addiction was minimized in several ways. Mrs. Henderson had been receiving the narcotic injections only a week. They had been given in response to complaints of severe pain. And on the previous day fewer injections had been given than on preceding days. The nurse then explained that Mrs. Henderson was very frightened of experiencing severe pain. Also, for several days at the beginning of hospitalization Mrs. Henderson had been frightened of the significance of her pain, fearing complications which did develop such as the hemorrhage that required a splenectomy. The nurse concluded by saying, "I think Mrs. Henderson is still afraid of severe pain. She may just want to know that the injections are available. In spite of your reassurances that she is doing well, I think she may also still fear that some other complications may arise. Perhaps we could try a tranquilizer three times a day to help her with her anxiety. This may reduce some of her pain. In addition, we could allow her to have the oral meperidine when she needs it. And, I think it would make her feel better if for the next few days she was allowed to have an injection of meperidine if the oral route doesn't relieve her pain. Sometimes she says her pain is severe. If you prescribe these drugs we can explain the plan to her and see how it works for about three days." These suggestions seemed reasonable to the physician, especially since gradual withdrawal of narcotics is one method of handling addiction if it does exist. He prescribed a tranquilizer and the oral and intramuscular meperidine. He limited the injections to twice a day for that day and the next two days. The nurse explained the new drug orders to Mrs. Henderson who expressed great relief that the injections were available. On that day Mrs. Henderson requested her second injection, but on each of the next two days she requested the injection only once. After that she relied on the oral meperidine for several days. Eventually she accepted the aspirin and no longer needed the tranquilizer. The nurse's understanding of the total situation contributed to a plan of analgesia that was acceptable to both patient and physician. If addiction was actually a possibility in this patient, it was averted without producing unnecessary panic in the patient or alarm in the physician.

The nurse contributes to the prevention of addiction in at least two ways. First, she may reduce the dosage and/or frequency of giving narcotics by using various pain relief measures in addition to narcotics. Secondly, her assessment of the patient's response to the narcotic and of the intensity of pain he experiences may prevent overly medicating the patient.

The comment is sometimes made that addiction in the terminally ill patient is of little concern. Assisting the dying patient to remain as comfortable as possible is a priority. However, the indiscriminate use of narcotics may have unfortunate results. Sometimes addiction makes it more difficult for the dying patient to manage his feelings (Gonda). And if the patient becomes addicted early in his illness, narcotics may be less effective toward the end when pain is even more severe. Therefore, as is true for all patients, other pain relief measures should be employed. This may delay the time when narcotics are needed, enhance the effectiveness of narcotics when they are employed, and decrease the dosage and frequency of narcotics. Yet, if pain relief cannot be achieved without narcotic addiction, terminal illness is the one circumstance in which this is allowed to happen.

Administering placebos. The term "placebo" is derived from a Latin word meaning "I shall please." This suggests that perhaps the first deliberate and conscious usage of the placebo was for the purpose of pleasing the patient who was asking for remedies or treatments that were unavailable, of no benefit, or possibly harmful. More recently the placebo has been used as a control in drug research. The effectiveness of a particular medication is evaluated by comparing it with an inert preparation called a placebo. As a result of these studies the placebo has become associated with inert oral and parenteral substances such as the "sugar pill" and saline injections. This brief history of the placebo accounts for the evolution of several among many misconceptions about the placebo. It is the purpose of this section both to correct some of the erroneous ideas surrounding the placebo and to suggest appropriate nursing activities related to its use.

To begin with, placebos do much more than "please" the patient. Also, they are not restricted to inert substances given as medication, although this is the most common form. A placebo may be defined as any medical treatment (medication or procedure, including surgery) that produces an effect in a patient because of its implicit or explicit therapeutic intent, and not because of its specific nature (physical or chemical properties). When a patient responds to a placebo in accordance with its intent he is said to be a placebo reactor for that occasion. His response is called a positive placebo response.

An incident described by a laboratory technician involving Mr. Grimes illustrates some aspects of this definition. Mr. Grimes had discomfort in his chest possibly associated with a cardiac problem. The laboratory technician, who had never before met Mr. Grimes, was sent to his hospital room to do an electrocardiogram (ECG). She entered the room with her equipment and pleasantly proceeded to introduce herself and to explain briefly the ECG. The patient asked no questions and appeared to understand the technician since he cooperated well with the procedure. After the ECG was completed and the technician was gathering her equipment to leave, the patient remarked, "This has helped me more than anything they've done for me so far. I wish you'd do it to that fellow over there; he seems to be having such a rough time." Obviously the technician's brief explanation was not sufficient for Mr. Grimes to understand that this was a diagnostic and not a therapeutic procedure. He seems to have assumed that the purpose of the ECG was to make him feel better. To him this purpose or intent was implicit in the ECG procedure; the intent of making him feel better certainly was not explicitly stated by the technician. He perceived an implicit intent of therapy and responded to it by feeling better. His response of feeling better is the placebo effect or positive placebo response. In this situation involving the ECG he is a placebo reactor. And, of course, the placebo was basically the ECG.

Placebo environment. Mr. Grimes' situation illustrates another important aspect of the placebo phenomenon—the placebo environment or the meaningful situation that is conducive to a positive placebo response. Although the ECG may be pointed to as the placebo, it is the situation in which it was presented and the multiple characteristics of the procedure itself that undoubtedly produced a placebo environment for Mr. Grimes. It is impossible to know which aspects of the placebo environment were the more significant ones to Mr. Grimes, but the following description probably includes them: Mr. Grimes was present in the hospital for the purpose of seeking assistance with his chest discomfort when someone came to his bedside, talked with him about a procedure that related to his chest discomfort, performed a series of tasks associated with his body, remained at his bedside about ten minutes, asked him to lie still for a while, directed attention to him, and used unfamiliar and probably awesome equipment. Four of the stimuli associated with a placebo environment are present in this situation. Some of these stimuli were alluded to in the definition of a placebo but they require further discussion.

First, the "treatment," as it was perceived by Mr. Grimes, was elaborate and convincing. Essentially it simply made sense to him that the ECG procedure would be effective in relieving his discomfort. He believed in it. This is not difficult to understand considering that the ECG equipment is relatively large, composed of many parts, and rather mysterious and complicated to the layman. The extent to which any treatment is convincing is determined by the individual upon whom it is performed. But as a general rule the more effective placebos are the ones with the greatest stimulus impact. For example, intravenous placebos are more effective than intramuscular ones, and bitter-tasting pills are more effective than pleasant ones.

Secondly, the person performing the procedure apparently was perceived by Mr. Grimes as being a trustworthy expert. Reactions to a placebo are significantly affected by cues the patient receives about the person performing the treatment. Undoubtedly the confidence, skill and expertise of this experienced technician contributed to convincing Mr. Grimes of her knowledge and competence.

Thirdly, the ECG itself and the verbal communications of the technician focused Mr. Grimes' attention upon the symptom being "treated." To obtain a positive placebo response it is almost essential that the patient be aware of the symptom that is to be altered.

The fourth aspect of the placebo environment is the communication of the intent of the placebo. Ordinarily this intent takes the form of an explicit verbal communication. For example, when a placebo is given for pain relief, the patient is told that it will relieve his pain. Sometimes included in the verbal communication are more convincing statements such as the treatment being a new breakthrough or being unusually potent. Of course, an implicit suggestion of the purpose of the placebo is often equally effective, as it was with Mr. Grimes. In studies on pain relief with placebos, the mere fact that an injection is given in response to a pain complaint is usually sufficient implicit suggestion to obtain a placebo response. Suggestion, either implicit or explicit, of the purpose of the placebo is a powerful and significant aspect of the placebo environment. This is demonstrated by the remarkable results of one study of 48 patients experiencing steady wound pain. Of these patients, 27 were told they were to receive a wonderful new drug that would completely relieve their pain. They received intravenous saline and one third reported pain relief. The other 21 patients were told they were to receive an injection of a new drug that was not very effective, but if it did not work they would receive an injection one hour later that would certainly relieve their pain. They were given morphine first and then saline, both intravenously. Seventeen reported pain relief from the morphine, but four reported no improvement or an increase in pain. These four patients account for less than 20 percent of the group, but it is highly interesting that morphine did not relieve their pain when they were told it was not very effective. What is even more astounding is that these four patients reported complete pain relief one hour later when saline was given intravenously (Keats).

This study not only illustrates the significance of suggestion in obtaining a positive placebo response, but also indicates that suggestion may counteract the effects of known pharmacological agents. Indeed, whatever is involved in the placebo phenomenon is applicable to all types of treatment and may either increase or decrease the effectiveness of proven treatments such as morphine. Every treatment has its placebo aspects, and the placebo effect cannot be avoided regardless of the treatment. Given the fact that the placebo effect exists, it is up to the nurse to capitalize on it. Other sections of this book cover the utilization of certain aspects of the placebo environment, such as suggestion, with all pain-relief measures. The use of these will not be repeated here because in this section we are concerned primarily with the usage of placebos *per se*.

Effects of placebos. Pain relief is not the only purpose for which a placebo may be used, nor is it the only effect that may result when the placebo is used for pain relief. Placebos have been used effectively to increase appetite, to induce sleep, to treat bleeding ulcers, to increase sexual desire, to decrease nausea, to relieve allergies, to remove skin blemishes and to lower blood pressure, to mention only a few. When placebos relieve pain they do so in a manner very similar to analgesics. The pattern of analgesia for the placebo often exhibits a time of onset, peak effect and duration comparable to analgesics such as morphine and aspirin. Side effects and toxic reactions also occur in response to placebos. These range from minor ones such as nasal stuffiness, dizziness and diarrhea to serious ones such as addiction and anaphylactoid reactions.

Placebo responses, whether they are the intended ones or the side effects of the intended ones, are not imaginary. Neither are they restricted to subjective reports by the individual. In the cases cited above, objective measures indicated that blood pressure did decrease, skin blemishes did disappear, and the reported decrease in nausea coincided with the resumption of gastric motor activity. Objective measures have also revealed placebo responses about which the individual receiving the placebo had no knowledge whatever. These responses included eosinophilia and a reduction in the concentration of serum lipoproteins. Thus, the patient may respond to a placebo with objectively measurable physiological changes over which he could have no direct, conscious control because he knows nothing about them (Wolf).

Not all patients will receive pain relief from a placebo, but this is true of all pain relief measures. There is no pain therapy (except one that produces loss of consciousness) that will relieve pain in all patients all the time. It is estimated that placebos will result in pain relief in about one third of the general patient population (Loan and Dundee, 1967b). This estimate is subject to several qualifications. The degree of pain relief may range from slight to complete, may be greater or less than that achieved by an analgesic, and may or may not be accompanied by side effects similar to those of an analgesic. Further, some patients will tend to be constant placebo reactors, defined as those who almost always react favorably to placebos. Others will be occasional placebo reactors, those who react positively to placebos only under certain conditions. Placebo reactors can be identified only by psychological testing such as the Rorschach inkblot test (Lasagna, *et al.*, 1954). On the basis of such tests the placebo reactor is often characterized as dependent, anxious, low in ego strength, low in self-sufficiency (Walike and Meyer), uncritically respectful of authority, unrealistic in life goals, immature, cooperative and neurotic (Liberman). While some of these attributes may not be considered desirable, the reader should realize that they are not easily observed. In no way do these attributes suggest that the placebo reactor tends to be an unlikeable person. The wide variation in the degree and occurrence of positive placebo responses coupled with the inability to identify a placebo reactor through ordinary observation makes it almost impossible to predict whether or not a placebo response will occur in a particular patient at a particular time.

Placebos in nursing practice. Thus far the discussion has focused on orienting the reader to a broad concept of the placebo phenomenon. Now we will turn to a consideration of nursing practice in relation to the usage of placebos for pain relief. Three topics will be covered: (1) the nurse's contribution to the interpretation of a patient's positive placebo response, (2) situations in which the nurse may suggest the usage of a placebo, and (3) the nursing activities associated with a physician's prescription of a placebo.

To contribute to the interpretation of a pain relief response following the administration of a placebo intended for pain relief, the nurse must realize that a true placebo response differs from other responses. Also, she must understand some of the possible mechanisms underlying the true placebo response. In other words, the nurse should be able to assess whether or not a true placebo response has occurred. If it has occurred she should know what it may or may not mean about the patient and his pain. For example, a patient may report pain relief after he has been given an injection of saline and told that the injection is for pain relief. There are at least four possible reasons for the report of pain relief. Only one of these possibilities is the true placebo response.

First, pain relief following a placebo may be due to measures other than the placebo. If other pain relief measures such as distraction or positioning were used at about the same time the placebo was administered, the pain relief may be a result of these and not the placebo. Further, if the patient has been receiving analgesics, he may be experiencing pain relief or pain control from their cumulative effects. When a potent analgesic such as morphine or meperidine is administered over a long period of time, a level of analgesia may be established that lasts for 24 to 72 hours after the last dose (Batterman). Such a patient may request an analgesic at a certain time out of habit or for the purpose of preventing an increase in pain. If a placebo is given, the absence of an increase in pain may be erroneously attributed to the placebo when it actually may be due to the cumulative effects of an analgesic.

Second, pain relief may be related to the spontaneous fluctuations in pain intensity that occur in the normal course of the particular disease. Many types of pain, especially chronic pain, increase and decrease in intensity from hour to hour in the absence of any form of pain relief measures. In other words, if the placebo had not been given the pain relief may have occurred anyway.

Thirdly, the patient may deliberately and consciously fake pain relief. We usually thank people for gifts we do not like simply because we are grateful for the kindness. Similarly the patient with pain may try to thank those who attempt to help him. He may do this by telling them that he feels better. Or, perhaps the patient simply wants to be what he thinks others consider a "good" patient. He cooperates with all that is asked of him and responds as he thinks he is expected to respond.

Fourthly, if the preceding three possibilities can be ruled out and if pain relief follows more than one administration of a placebo, it is likely that the patient is making a true placebo response. Most of the time in actual practice a placebo is substituted for a drug the patient has been receiving. For example, if the patient has been getting morphine injections, saline injections are substituted. If he has been receiving oral codeine, capsules of the same appearance containing sugar are substituted. The patient's response to the placebo is compared to his response to the medication replaced by the placebo. This comparison may reveal that the effectiveness of the placebo is the same as, greater than or less than the medication it replaces. As long as the patient reports a significant degree of pain relief, even if this is less than that caused by the original medication, the result is considered a true placebo response. Further, a positive and true placebo response will not necessarily occur every time a placebo is administered, just as pain relief will not occur after every morphine injection.

Sometimes the decision to place the patient on placebos is a rather hasty one. The decision may be based on the favorable results of a single administration of a placebo. Knowing that in addition to a true placebo response there are at least three possible reasons for pain relief to follow a placebo, the nurse can encourage health team members to evaluate more thoroughly the effectiveness of the placebo.

Various mechanisms have been suggested to explain the occurrence of a positive and true placebo response. The three that will be mentioned here are reduced anxiety, classical conditioning, and self-judgment of suppression of avoidance or escape responses. The reader will note that these same mechanisms are used to explain the effectiveness of many other pain-relief measures. This suggests that the placebo phenomenon has much in common with other pain therapies. In short, a positive placebo response is probably produced by processes rather similar to those responsible for the pain relief following various other measures. This is an important point and will be emphasized in the discussion of the three mechanisms underlying a positive and true placebo response.

First, as we have mentioned many times before, a decrease in anxiety about pain results in pain relief. Apparently placebos contribute to pain relief by reducing anxiety. The placebo reactor is willing and able to reduce his anxiety either through the ministrations of someone he trusts to help him or through the stimulus of something he associates with pain relief. It is interesting that placebos rarely produce pain relief when anxiety is not present or is kept high by other factors (Sternbach, 1968). However, this appears to be equally true of other pain relief measures such as morphine and hypnosis. For example, although morphine dependably relieves pathological pain, it does not dependably relieve experimental pain unless anxiety is produced in the experimental situation (Beecher, 1966). Often the comment is made that the patient reacts positively to the placebo because he is anxious. This is true, but it is also true of the patient who obtains pain relief from morphine or hypnosis. Therefore, one must conclude that a major difference between the placebo reactor and the patient who receives pain relief from such measures as morphine is largely the manner in which anxiety is reduced. The patient who requires morphine for pain relief relies upon a pharmacological substance for anxiety reduction. The patient who requires only a placebo relies on environmental stimuli such as the people and/or the procedure itself for anxiety reduction.

The second mechanism related to a positive placebo response is classical conditioning. The reader will recall that this mechanism also at least partially explains the effectiveness of pain relief measures such as the Lamaze method. Classical conditioning probably also underlies the occurrence of immediate pain relief from an injection of morphine. When classical conditioning is thought to underlie a pain relief response, it may be explained thus: whatever stimulus or set of stimuli has been associated in the past with pain relief will tend to produce pain relief in the future. For example, if injections of morphine have relieved a patient's pain, the stimuli associated with the administration of an injection may acquire the property of inducing pain relief. As a result the patient may receive pain relief from the placebo injection of saline if he believes it is morphine. In fact, it apparently is not always necessary for him to possess the higher cognitive ability to evaluate the injection as being morphine since placebo responses occur in rats and possibly infants. Placebo responses have been demonstrated in rats by associating saline and scopolamine injections. Originally scopolamine depressed lever-pressing behavior in the rats and saline alone did not. Eventually an injection of saline was sufficient to depress the lever-pressing behavior (Herrnstein). With regard to infants, an acquaintance of this author reports that she accidentally administered vitamins instead of an analgesic to her ten-month-old daughter who had otitis media. This occurred in the middle of the night and the mother did not cuddle the infant or administer any other pain relief measures. Yet, the infant stopped crying and went to sleep. This was the same behavior that had followed the use of the analgesic on previous nights. Among the possible explanations for this infant's behavior is that a positive placebo response occurred. Perhaps the baby had been conditioned to obtain pain relief either from the presence of the mother or from the mother administering an oral substance in a medicine dropper.

From these examples we may conclude that in some cases conditioning is firmly established. Conditioning may lead to a placebo response in the absence of any intellectual evaluation of the placebo by the patient. In other instances the patient may require or have relied upon the verbal stimulus of being told that the treatment is for the purpose of pain relief. In other words, some patients may be conditioned to experience pain relief from the stimuli of a particular treatment such as an injection or a pill. Others will be conditioned to the stimuli of both a certain treatment and the verbal statement of its purpose. Still others may be conditioned only to the verbal statement. If the latter is true, then a placebo response may follow any treatment that is accompanied by a verbal statement of its purpose or effectiveness. In this case it will not matter whether or not the patient previously has received the treatment or something similar.

A third mechanism that may underlie a true and positive placebo response is concerned with the notion of self-observation as a source of pain perception. According to this theory, a person uses his own overt behavioral responses to a noxious stimulus to evaluate the intensity of the pain. When a person voluntarily or involuntarily suppresses escape or avoidance responses, he considers this behavior in himself to mean that the pain is less intense. When a patient receives a placebo he may suppress these escape responses because of instructions, suggestions, conditioning, or decreased anxiety. Regardless of the reason, the patient observes himself and notes that he has not tried to avoid the noxious stimuli. He then tends to decide in favor of a decreased intensity of pain (Bandler, Madaras and Bem). The reader may remember that this theory may also explain the effectiveness of pain-relief measures such as relaxation.

In addition to these three mechanisms that may underlie a positive placebo response, other principles of achieving pain relief are involved. These include resolution of cognitive dissonance, the production of behaviors incompatible with pain, and the use of what the patient believes will relieve pain.

The placebo phenomenon is complex, but it is not magic. It can be explained on the basis of scientific principles and theories that also explain other pain relief measures. And certainly, the pain relief of a true and positive placebo response is as genuine and real as any other pain relief. But old ideas and beliefs sometimes die hard. So it is with the placebo. When a patient receives pain relief from a placebo, there are usually some health team members who draw two erroneous conclusions. In an atmosphere of knowing smiles, a little laughter, and nodding heads it is clear, even if it is never spoken, that the patient is viewed as some sort of weird, crazy, or neurotic individual whose pain does not originate with any physical or physiological stimulus. It is thought that he is either deliberately faking the pain or "just thinks he has pain." A positive placebo response is not proof of malingering. And, according to the definition of pain set forth in this book, *if a patient "thinks" he has pain, he does have pain.* Considering the wealth of research on placebos, it is amazing that some people still believe that a positive placebo response means there is no physical stimulus for the pain. Studies show that pain relief following a placebo is reported by 35 to 40 percent of patients suffering acute postoperative pain or chronic pain from cancer (Beecher, 1959). Can we say that these patients did not "really" feel pain or that the surgical incision or malignant mass did not exist? The only reasonable conclusion is that some mentally healthy persons exposed to intense noxious stimuli will receive pain relief from a placebo.

Clearly, it is a gross injustice to the patient to believe that his positive placebo response means he is a neurotic who has no cause to feel pain in the first place. *A much more accurate conclusion about the placebo reactor is that he very much wants to be relieved of his pain and that he trusts something or someone, perhaps the nurse, to help him obtain pain relief.* This is hardly a matter deserving of laughter. To this writer, misunderstanding of such a patient is one of the saddest and most lamentable occurrences in all of health care.

Sammy, 19 years old, illustrates some of what may happen when a positive placebo response is evaluated incorrectly. Sammy was admitted to the hospital with renal failure. Eventually a left kidney transplant was performed, but was removed because of infection. A few weeks afterwards Sammy began complaining of moderate to severe pain on his left side somewhat below the surgical area. No cause for the pain could be determined, and it was tentatively decided that this was referred pain from the tender area of the previous incision. The complaints of pain persisted for about a week, and Sammy refused to ambulate because of the pain. Darvon was given orally for a few days but did not produce pain relief. The physician then ordered one dose of a placebo, 1 cc. of normal saline intramuscularly, for the next complaint of pain in the left side. This is a typical situation in which a placebo is ordered. The patient often has an extensive medical history and complains of pain persistently while no physiological basis can be found for the cause of the pain. Fifteen minutes after the placebo was administered to Sammy he reported considerable pain relief for the first time and fell asleep. After this no other placebos or analgesics were ordered, and the physician insisted that Sammy ambulate in spite of the pain.

This situation did not allow for a complete assessment of the effectiveness of the placebo since it was given only once. Sammy's report of pain relief may have been a true placebo response, but it also could have been mostly gratitude for someone finally doing something to help his pain. The fact that no other pain relief measures were ordered shows little sympathy or understanding of Sammy's situation and probably reflects an evaluation of Sammy as a neurotic or á faker. This occurrence of pain relief following a placebo seemed to be interpreted by the physician as meaning that Sammy had no reason to feel pain. This conclusion is unjustified regardless of whether or not a cause for the pain is ever found. One cannot escape the idea that such a conclusion represents the physician's belief that if pain exists he should be able to determine the cause. It would be wonderful if this were true, but medical science simply is not that advanced. However, in Sammy's case the cause was finally found, delayed somewhat because of the inaccurate conclusion that pain relief following a placebo indicates no physical stimulus for pain. Two weeks after the incident with the placebo a new physician assumed responsibility for Sammy's care. He ordered an x-ray of the area in which Sammy complained of pain. A fractured femur of several weeks duration was revealed. This was a spontaneous fracture due to osteoporosis caused by prednisone and other medications.

This situation would not have occurred if the health team members had understood the placebo phenomenon. A search for the cause of the pain would have continued. Analgesics and perhaps placebos would have been ordered. Other methods would have been used to alleviate anxiety and pain. Certainly the patient's pain would not have been ignored. And, if placebos had been ordered, they would not have been relied upon exclusively. Knowing that a positive placebo response reflects a motivation to obtain pain relief, the nurses would have continued or increased their efforts to assist the patient. The patient's trust in them would not have been interpreted as neurosis.

Although a placebo cannot be used to rule out a physical basis for pain or to diagnose neurosis or malingering, there are situations in which it may be appropriate for the nurse to suggest that a placebo be considered as one method of pain relief. However, the nurse should realize that the use of a placebo involves certain ethical and legal considerations. The physician, not the nurse, prescribes a placebo medication. For ethical reasons some physicians will refuse to use a placebo knowingly. Placebos are, after all, the major form of treatment employed by quacks. The conscientious physician does not casually make a decision to administer deliberately a treatment that has no known or proven therapeutic properties. Nevertheless, the nurse may suggest the use of placebos for pain relief in the following circumstances: (1) when the administration of certain drugs such as narcotics and steroids produce undesirable side effects or may possibly lead to addiction, (2) when a procedure cannot be done in the presence of an analgesic, or (3) when medications and procedures seem to be the only form of communication the patient understands.

The relief of chronic pain sometimes leads to the use of narcotics or steroids over a prolonged period of time. To control the occurrence of undesirable side effects or addiction, a placebo may be substituted for the medication. The placebo may be substituted for every administration of the medication or may be used intermittently. The latter is usually more effective since the continued use of the real drug at intervals maintains the conditioning of the patient. For example, in a patient with chronic pain, every other injection may be a placebo, alternated with morphine. If the patient makes a positive placebo response, this may be due to the conditioning established with the morphine. The conditioning is maintained by continuing the morphine at regular intervals. When a placebo is substituted for morphine or some other drug, it is possible that the placebo response will include some of the same side effects as the drug it replaces. Addiction may even occur. However, it is more likely that pain relief will occur without side effects or addiction. If undesirable effects do occur, they probably will be less severe than those associated with the drug for which the placebo is a substitute.

Occasionally the patient with pain undergoes procedures that cannot be performed accurately or effectively in the presence of analgesics. For example, the results of certain diagnostic tests that assess cardiac or brain function may be affected if the patient has received morphine prior to the test. If the patient must endure pain without an analgesic for a certain period of time prior to such a test, the nurse may suggest the use of a placebo only for this period of time.

There appears to be a certain type of patient whose anxiety increases the intensity of pain. Yet he seems unable to respond to interpersonal communications designed to reduce the anxiety. This type of patient may be characterized as relating to objects and not to people. He does not even seem to relate to himself; his insight about himself is quite limited. He often denies anxiety, insisting that he is not worried about anything. He complains frequently of pain but cannot be encouraged to discuss what his pain means to him. He is sometimes described as demanding and manipulative. He may refuse professional assistance from a psychiatrist or psychologist. Occasionally the patient is diagnosed as hysterical, not necessarily because his pain is thought to be hysterical pain but because he uses repression to handle anxiety and conflicts. With this type of patient, reducing his anxiety and expressing concern for him seem to be more readily achieved through the use of treatments. Often these treatments are medications for pain relief. Since the administration of medications to this patient may be one of the few forms of communication that effectively relieve his anxiety and pain, placebos may be substituted for drugs in an effort to maintain communication but prevent the dangers of excessive medication.

Miss Sterling, 32 years old, illustrates two of the situations in which it is appropriate to use placebos—to prevent the side effects and addiction associated with the continued administration of narcotics, and to communicate with the patient in a manner that is understood by the patient. Miss Sterling had a long and complicated medical history which, as mentioned previously, is typical of patients for whom placebos are considered. The medical history could not be viewed as accurate because Miss Sterling gave different information to different people. She variously reported, 16, 19 and 30 surgical operations in the pelvic area. But, any of these numbers is impressive and indicates the extent of her illnesses. This patient was known to have pathology sufficient to account for her reports of pain. Among other signs and symptoms she had severe hematuria and pyuria and a possibly malignant mass in the breast.

Miss Sterling was unable to benefit from any pain relief measures except injections. When the nurse tried to teach her to use distraction, Miss Sterling attempted to cooperate but finally said, "I don't think I can do it. I just can't concentrate on anything." When the nurse introduced breathing techniques, Miss Sterling said, "I don't think I want to try that. It's too complicated." Relaxation techniques were equally ineffective; Miss Sterling could not relax in spite of repeated attempts. Since there was ample reason to suspect that Miss Sterling was anxious about the meaning of her pain, the nurse attempted to explore this with her. The results were poor. Miss Sterling totally denied any anxiety or worry. For example, when the nurse asked how she felt about the possible mastectomy, Miss Sterling replied, "That's OK. I don't mind." All of the nurse's questions and comments were met with similar responses.

Miss Sterling continued to demand her analgesic at regular and frequent intervals. The analgesic was meperidine and chlorpromazine given intramuscularly at the same time in two injections. Miss Sterling had a history of drug abuse and it was decided that she should not continue to receive this amount of meperidine. Because measures other than injections did not provide pain relief and because of the danger of addiction in this patient with chronic pain of one sort or another, the nurse suggested alternating the two drugs with a placebo. Ascorbic acid, 1 cc. intramuscularly, was prescribed as the placebo. In appearance ascorbic acid is similar to the other drugs, and it produces a sensation comparable to the other drugs when injected. After each of the first three injections of the placebo Miss Sterling reported no pain relief. However, when the ascorbic acid was given in two injections, as were the other drugs, Miss Sterling reported complete pain relief. Rather than risk addiction or, as the other alternative, deprive this patient of her only means of pain relief, a placebo was successfully alternated with other drugs for the duration of her hospitalization.

Whenever a placebo is prescribed the nurse should obtain certain information from the physician and record it in the nursing care plan. Everyone who cares for the patient should know what the patient is to be told about the placebo; otherwise he may receive conflicting information and begin to suspect that he is receiving a placebo. This may be very upsetting to the patient since most patients believe, as do some health team members, that a placebo is given because no one believes he has pain.

The nurse should find out whether the placebo is supposed to represent a new drug or the same drug the patient has been receiving. If the latter, then every effort must be made to obtain a placebo that has the same appearance and taste or sensation upon injection. When the patient asks questions about the placebo, they should be answered in the same way they would be for the drugs the placebo replaces. If the placebo is supposed to be a new drug, the nurse should ask the physician the name by which the placebo is to be called and all of the characteristics it is supposed to have. For example, in discussing the "drug" with the patient and in answering his questions, the nurse may be expected to tell the patient the following: that it is a new and very effective drug called by the experimental name of ZQ-129, that it should relieve his pain within 15 minutes and last up to six hours, and that it may make him drowsy. This is, of course, largely a lie. If the nurse does not feel she can do this convincingly and in good conscience, she should not hesitate to ask someone else to administer the placebo. She may unwittingly convey her feelings to the patient and thereby impair the effect of the placebo.

The nurse also needs to know whether or not the physician ever plans to tell the patient he has received a placebo. Some physicians may choose to confront the patient with his positive placebo response for the purpose of helping the patient recognize and handle the anxiety that contributes to pain. The patient will need assistance in coping with this information. And the nurse may wish to refuse to give the placebo if she feels that her relationship with the patient will be destroyed when he learns that she administered the placebo.

Using waking-imagined analgesia. The patient's use of his imagination to decrease his perception of the intensity of pain is an ancient phenomenon. This method of dealing with pain has recently been rendered less elusive and more accessible to everyday nursing practice because some investigators have defined and described it. It is called waking-imagined analgesia (WIA). This may be defined as imagining a pleasant situation when a noxious stimulus is applied (Barber and Hahn). WIA is similar to distraction and is actually a form of distraction with one important difference. In distraction the patient focuses on enumerating or describing objects or events unrelated to the pain but occurring in the present or recalled from memory of past events. For example, the patient who uses distraction during a painful experience may describe a series of pictures, watch television, count spots on the ceiling, or recall the details of a vacation trip. In WIA the patient uses his imagination to deal with pain by trying to relive all of the sensations of a previous possibly pleasant experience. Rather than focusing only on a description of the experience, he tries to recreate within himself all the sensations associated with the experience. He imagines that the experience is happening again. With an active imagination, the body begins to respond as it did when the event occurred.

Sometimes there is a fine line between recalling an event and actually reliving it, but there is a difference. The reader may experience this difference by doing two simple things. First, describe to yourself how you prepare a lemon for eating, how you hold it when you eat it, and how you place your mouth on it to suck or take a bite. Secondly, try to imagine how a lemon tastes. This simple exercise may reveal several things about the difference between WIA and distraction and about how active your imagination is. Did your mouth begin to water during the description of eating a lemon? If it did, you have an active imagination and you see that a description may become more than just a distraction—the thin line may be crossed and the imagination may be activated, causing the body to respond with salivation. On the other hand, your mouth may not have watered until you began to imagine the taste of a lemon, demonstrating that distraction and imagination may be two entirely different experiences. Imagination is a step beyond the thought processes of distraction. Imagination involves a more total response that includes both thought processes and bodily processes or sensations.

When a patient uses WIA, what does he imagine when a noxious stimulus is applied? In the strictest sense of the use of WIA, he should imagine something that produces analgesia for the particular painful sensation. In other words, he uses his imagination to interpret a specific painful sensation as being a sensation other than painful. He does this by substituting some previously experienced pleasant or nonpainful sensation for the painful sensation. For example, if a patient is to have a painful soak to his leg, he may imagine that his leg is soaking in cool, soothing water while he is sitting at the side of a swimming pool on a warm day. Or, if the patient is having a lumbar puncture, he may imagine that someone is giving him a relaxing back rub on his lower back. The soaking in cool water and the back rub are examples of substituting a pleasant sensation for a painful sensation. A common example of substituting a nonpainful but not especially pleasant sensation for a painful sensation is the imagination of insensitivity of the painful area. For instance, the patient with the painful leg soak might imagine that the leg has "fallen asleep" from decreased circulation and is now insensitive to stimuli. In all these examples we are assuming that the patient has previously experienced the sensation substituted for pain. It is far easier for the patient to imagine a back rub, for example, if he has experienced one. Similarly, with the lemon exercise suggested to the reader, salivation would have been unlikely if the reader had never eaten a lemon.

In a broader sense WIA may involve imagining pleasant, relaxing, or perhaps exciting events of a more general nature. These more general types of events involve sensations, but the sensations are not specific substitutes for a particular area of pain. An example of this type of WIA is presented in the section on providing other sensory input. The nurse suggested to Mr. Wiley that during his myelogram he use his imagination as one form of distraction. Mr. Wiley chose to imagine sexual intercourse with his wife. He considered this pleasant and interesting, capable of distracting him during pain. The bodily sensations accompanying sexual intercourse did not permit Mr. Wiley to interpret the painful sensations of the myelogram as other than painful. The sexual sensations merely distracted him from the painful sensations. Since this type of WIA is quite similar to distraction, it is usually presented to the patient as a form of distraction. For a further discussion of distraction the reader is referred to the section on providing other sensory input.

We will return now to a discussion of the form of WIA that involves the imagination of a pleasant or nonpainful sensation as a substitute for the painful sensation, allowing the interpretation of the painful sensation as nonpainful. Just as some patients naturally, without suggestions from the nurse, use distraction to deal with pain, so, too, may some patients use WIA on their own. To distract himself from his pain a patient may deliberately watch television or initiate a conversation. The naturally occuring usage of WIA seems to be less common, but some people report that they use it. For example, one patient said that by imagining the sensation of brushing his teeth he was able to tolerate dental drilling without a local anesthetic. Another patient revealed that she tolerated the first stage of labor without anesthesia or analgesia by imagining sexual intercourse. She even reported having several orgasms! It is not uncommon for patients to report a similarity between the second stage of labor and sexual intercourse and/or a bowel movement, but this patient was referring to the first stage of labor. Apparently she imagined the sensations of sexual intercourse and interpreted the sensations of the uterine contractions as sexual ones.

The effective use of WIA is probably limited to a smaller percentage of the patient population than some other pain relief measures such as distraction. This possibility has already been suggested by the fact that fewer people seem naturally to employ WIA. In addition, WIA cannot be imposed upon the patient; he must be willing and able to use his imagination. Distraction, on the other hand, can be more or less imposed upon the patient by almost making him answer questions. And, distraction can be an effective pain relief measure even when the patient states that he does not believe distraction will help him. But it is unlikely that a patient would even try to use his imagination if he did not believe it would be beneficial. Further, WIA has much in common with hypnosis. Therefore, its usage may be subject to the same limitations as hypnotic analgesia. WIA is believed by some to be essentially the same as hypnotic analgesia but without the accompanying hypnotic induction and trance. WIA has been reported to be as effective as hypnotic analgesia when it is used on good hypnotic subjects (those who score high on suggestibility tests). Although about 90 percent of the population can enter the first stage of hypnosis (relaxation), hypnotic anesthesia or analgesia seems to be obtained only in the second stage, or cataleptic state, of hypnosis. Estimates of the persons in the population able to experience hypnotic analgesia range from five to 25 percent (Barber; Barber and Hahn; Kroger). If the effective usage of WIA is limited to good hypnotic subjects, then it will be useful with relatively fewer patients than some other pain relief measures.

Since patients rarely receive suggestibility tests, the nurse will not know whether or not a particular patient is a good hypnotic subject who would benefit from WIA. She must simply apply WIA on a trial-and-error basis. If the patient reports that he naturally and successfully used WIA in a previous situation, this may be a good indication that he will benefit from it for a current painful experience. But, WIA also may be successful if he has never before used it. Since children above the age of three years may be good hypnotic subjects, the nurse should not limit the usage of WIA to adults. Many children are very susceptible to suggestion and have excellent imaginations.

The nurse's approach to the use of WIA is similar to that for any other pain relief measure. Basically, she explains the technique and finds out whether or not the patient wishes to try it. However, there are certain important aspects of the method of instructing the patient in WIA. When the nurse introduces WIA to the patient, she should include the following: statements and questions that motivate the patient to try to use his imagination; positive statements about the effectiveness of WIA and about the patient's ability to use his imagination successfully; no mention of the word pain, but use of other words such as discomfort; and indirect suggestions of analgesia (to avoid defining the situation as one in which pain is inevitable or expected) (Barber and Hahn). The suggestion of analgesia may be insensitivity of the painful part or substitution of a non-painful sensation for a painful sensation. When the latter is used and when there are major variations in the painful sensations, the nurse may need to suggest the substitution of several different nonpainful sensations. This is illustrated in the following example, which also incorporates the important aspects of instruction in WIA and includes the use of various other approaches to pain relief such as involving the patient in a decision about the effectiveness of the pain relief measure and using touch and relaxation through imagination.

Mrs. Hardy's physician informed her he would do a bone marrow aspiration of the sternum in about two hours. The nurse explained the procedure to Mrs. Hardy and included a description of the three variations in the sensations of the procedure: the stinging as the local anesthetic is injected, the pressure as the needle enters the bone, and the discomfort during aspiration. To begin to motivate Mrs. Hardy to use her imagination and to suggest that she would be successful, the nurse said, "It seems to me that you're a creative person. Do you have a good imagination when you want to use it?" When Mrs. Hardy replied affirmatively, the nurse continued, "If you think about what's happening during the procedure you may find it uncomfortable, but if you use your imagination you will not be bothered by it. It all depends upon your willingness to use your imagination. I'm sure you could do this well. If you're willing to try it, I'll explain what to do. Do you want to try?" These comments were designed to increase Mrs. Hardy's motivation to use her imagination, to express confidence in her ability to use her imagination, and to engage her in a decision about using the technique.

Since Mrs. Hardy wanted to hear more about the technique, the nurse said, "Lie down here in bed with this pillow under your back as it will be during the procedure. Now look up at the ceiling and focus on one point. Begin to try to imagine that you are lying in a very soft bed and are very relaxed. When the procedure begins, imagine that someone is placing a cool lotion on your chest and is beginning to rub the middle of your chest. If you want to, I'm sure you can imagine this. Imagine that the rubbing starts lightly with a pleasant tickling sensation. Then the rubbing becomes harder and harder just like a good strong back rub when your muscles are tired. Imagine that the muscles in your chest are becoming more and more relaxed with the harder rubbing. Keep imagining how pleasant and relaxing it is to be rubbed." These instructions attempted to account for two of the impending painful sensations—tickling was substituted for the injection of the anasthetic and hard rubbing for the pressure of entering the bone.

Further discussion with Mrs. Hardy revealed that she understood the instructions and did not feel that she wanted them repeated. The nurse then asked, "Do you want to try to use your imagination in this way during the procedure?" Mrs. Hardy replied, "I don't think so." She went on to explain, "It's interesting and it might work, but it doesn't make sense to me. I've always used distraction and tried not to think about the pain. It just doesn't make sense to me to focus on the pain and try to call it something else. I'd rather not pay any attention to the pain. Would you help me use a distraction?" Naturally, the nurse complied with the patient's wishes and Mrs. Hardy effectively used distraction during the bone marrow aspiration.

It is understandable that Mrs. Hardy would want to rely upon a pain relief measure that had been successful for her in the past, but her comments about WIA deserve our attention. Clinical experience in the use of WIA is limited at this time, so all refusals to use it are worthy of special consideration. Mrs. Hardy's reasons for refusing to use WIA are typical of the comments made by others who refuse WIA. As Mrs. Hardy indicated, this form of WIA tends to focus the patient's attention on the area of discomfort. This will increase the perceived intensity of pain unless the imagination is powerful enough to substitute a non-painful sensation. Mrs. Hardy had never consciously used WIA, and she implied that the technique was foreign to her coping style. This suggests that even those patients who could use WIA successfully may require some practice with it. The need for practice is also supported by the fact that hypnotic analgesia, which is similar to WIA, often requires several hypnotic sessions and sometimes weeks or months of practice.

Two examples of the successful use of WIA provide additional clinical data about this relatively new technique. In the first example a patient, Miss Cahill, complained of a sore throat and would not eat because of the discomfort. The nurse asked her to describe the sensations in her throat. The patient's description included the phrases "like a hand around my throat, applying pressure" and "pressing and constricting." The nurse suggested to Miss Cahill that she imagine the discomfort was actually someone's hand placed snugly around her throat. Miss Cahill agreed to try this and was able to eat.

In the second example, Mrs. Tindel was hospitalized for diagnosis of a genitourinary problem. She also had a ten-year history of vascular headaches. On the third day of hospitalization she complained of a vascular headache. She described the pain as intense throbbing localized on her forehead above her left eye. The medication Mrs. Tindel usually took for these headaches had not been ordered by the physician. During the hour that Mrs. Tindel had to wait for the physician to prescribe a medication, the nurse tried several pain-relief measures. Mrs. Tindel was willing to try them all, including cutaneous stimulation, relaxation, rhythmic breathing and distraction. None of these worked for more than about ten minutes. The nurse then explained WIA. She suggested that Mrs. Tindel substitute for the throbbing a nonpainful sensation of her choice. The nurse was called away at this point, but a few hours later after the headache had subsided with medication, Mrs. Tindel discussed her reactions to WIA. Mrs. Tindel told the nurse, "That business of imagining another sensation in place of the pain—it's interesting. I've never heard of that before, but it worked just as well as the other things we tried. I guess it worked for about ten minutes. At first I didn't know what to imagine. I tried to think of a ball inside my head causing pressure, but that didn't work at all. Then I thought about a band around my head that was pressing something hard on my left forehead. That helped a little, but the idea of a tight band seemed to make my muscles tense. Then I just imagined that someone was pressing the tips of his fingers against my forehead, and that worked." Mrs. Tindel paused and laughingly added, "but I couldn't think of a good reason why someone would be doing that (pressing the forehead with the finger tips). At that point it stopped working. But I'm going to try it again sometime."

In both of these examples of the successful use of WIA the patients externalized the source of pain and imagined the less uncomfortable sensation of pressure. Possibly this reduced their anxiety about the pain and in turn decreased the perceived intensity of pain. Perhaps some of the anxiety associated with pain was the feeling that their own bodies were out of control. Imagining that the cause of pain was outside the body may have relieved this anxiety. Anxiety may have been further reduced by labeling the sensation pressure instead of pain, or "sore" or "throbbing." The word "pressure" probably elicits less anxiety than some pain-related terms. Also, it may have been easier to imagine pressure than some other sensation such as coolness, since pressure more closely resembled the painful sensation. From these examples, we may hypothesize that one successful way of using WIA is to assist the patient to imagine that the source of pain is external to his body and to imagine a sensation that is similar to the discomfort but more acceptable (and not necessarily very pleasant).

In addition to anxiety reduction, several other mechanisms or principles may be involved in the production of pain relief through WIA. The usual behavioral response to pain is to focus on the pain, but in the case of WIA, the patient focuses on a sensation other than pain. If focusing on a sensation other than pain causes the patient to suppress avoidance responses, he behaves in another way that is incompatible with pain responses. Suppression of avoidance responses may also cause him to evaluate the intensity of pain as being less. For a discussion of the mechanism of using self-observation of suppressed escape responses as a source of pain perception, the reader is referred to the sections on promoting rest and relaxation and administering placebos.

When a patient uses WIA, other health team members should be informed of ways they may assist the patient and of certain factors that may lessen the patient's ability to use WIA. The word "pain" should not be used. Rather, discomfort should be referred to as the sensation the patient is trying to imagine such as coolness, numbness or pressure. If the patient begins to feel discomfort, he should be reminded of the sensation he was imagining. For example, the nurse or physician might say, "Remember the pressure. Someone is just pressing there." But, when the patient is quite engrossed in imagining, he probably will not want to be interrupted.

Decreasing noxious stimuli. There are many ways the nurse may alter the source of pain to decrease noxious stimuli. Several have already been discussed, such as the administration of medications that cure or control the disease process that causes the pain and the use of relaxation techniques to decrease pain from pressure or muscle spasms. The method the nurse uses to decrease noxious stimuli depends upon the patient's particular pathology. Since there are a huge variety of disease conditions, each one affecting various patients differently, the discussion must be limited to an almost random assortment of methods.

As mentioned in Chapter 3, certain environmental conditions may cause or increase pain. If a patient has no dressings covering his second-degree burns,the nurse should carefully avoid all drafts: even a very mild air current will stimulate the exposed nerve endings and produce pain. The nurse may caution certain patients about high altitudes. Ascent should be slow to prevent a crisis in the patient with sickle cell anemia or to prevent a migraine headache in a person with a history of vascular headaches. If the patient experiences eye pain or chest pain from air pollution, the nurse may suggest the use of an air conditioner. However, she should warn the patient that the effectiveness of the air conditioner in removing the offending pollutant will depend upon the type of filter used. The nurse may suggest to a patient with chronic lung disease that he avoid visiting or living in those cities with severe air pollution problems.

Pain on movement is associated with many pathological conditions ranging from surgical wounds to arthritis, and is frequently more difficult to relieve than steady pain. Often the patient has constant but tolerable discomfort that increases considerably with certain motor activities. Sometimes the injured area must be exercised to prevent complications such as contractures of the surrounding muscles. In other cases, pain on movement occurs in the course of simple activities of daily living such as eating and changing positions. Or, the pain occurs because of prescribed activities such as coughing and ambulating to prevent respiratory and circulatory complications. When painful activities are necessary but are not for the specific purpose of exercising the injured area, there are several ways the nurse may assist the patient to decrease the noxious stimuli associated with movement.

Usually the patient can tell the nurse which types of movement are especially painful, and the nurse can help the patient to avoid them. But, when painful movements cannot be avoided completely, the nurse may suggest some supportive measures that minimize them. To do this she must understand what is causing the pain. Common causes of pain on movement are related to pressure on the injured area, contraction of injured muscles, or displacement of or traction on a body part. Pressure on an injured area may be due to adjacent organs or the contraction of surrounding muscles. For example, upper abdominal pain of visceral origin may be increased by the pressure of the diaphragm. To decrease this source of noxious stimuli the nurse may suggest that the patient pull his shoulders backward and hold his arms away from his body to allow for lateral expansion of the lungs. If the pain is increased by contraction of surrounding muscles, the nurse may suggest splinting the area. She may also recommend positioning that minimizes the use of those muscles.

Since splinting supports the injured area with less usage of surrounding muscles, it will also alleviate the painful contraction of injured muscles. In addition, the nurse may help the patient substitute other muscle power for the activities that ordinarily involve the injured muscles. For example, if the patient has an abdominal incision, he can be taught to get out of bed by using his leg and arm muscles instead of his abdominal muscles. Prior to assisting a particular patient with pain to move, the nurse may wish to determine for herself which activities involve injured muscles or muscles surrounding the injured area. A useful method of learning this is for the nurse to place adhesive tape on herself in the area of the patient's pain. For instance, if the patient has an incision, the nurse can assume a position that places no strain on that area. Then she can place a strip of adhesive tape on herself in the region corresponding to the patient's incision. On either side of the incision and perpendicular to it she can place several more strips of tape. With the tape in place she can try different methods of sitting, walking and getting in and out of bed. When the tape pulls her skin she will know that the activity probably will be painful for the patient.

The pain associated with traction on or displacement of a body part may also be alleviated by assuming certain positions or using other muscles. An example of this is the spinal headache. This headache is apparently due to drainage of cerebrospinal fluid, causing displacement of and traction on the contents of the cranium. As a result, the patient experiences a headache when he stands up. Gravity displaces the brain and places traction on the various pain-sensitive structures that anchor it to the cranium (Wolff and Wolf). Lying flat in bed without a pillow usually alleviates discomfort. When the patient must assume an erect position, some of the noxious stimuli will be decreased if the nurse instructs him to flex or extend his neck.

Some of the noxious stimuli associated with painful procedures and wound dressings may be decreased by a few simple measures. Certain procedures and most dressing changes involve the use of adhesive tape, which may be a constant source of minor discomfort to the patient since it irritates the skin and pulls tiny hairs. Whenever possible a binder or an elastic, nonadhesive material should be used to hold the dressing in place and provide support to the area. Or, if dressings are done daily and support is not necessary, adhesive tape may be used if it is not removed daily. This may be accomplished if the tape adheres to the skin on either side of the wound but does not adhere to the dressing. On each side the strap of tape is doubled back on itself so that it does not stick to the dressing. The straps are held together over the dressing by safety pins, gauze strips or rubber bands. To avoid further irritation when the tape is removed, it may be moistened with warm water. The adhesive substance that remains on the skin may be removed with mineral oil or olive oil rather than the more caustic benzine or alcohol.

To decrease the duration of pain caused by dressings or other procedures, the nurse should work as quickly as possible as long as speed does not result in more pain. The nurse should also remember that pain intensity is not generally increased by the summation of neural impulses from noxious stimulation at different sites. For example, if a large wound must be packed, the pain of packing will not be any greater if several areas are packed at one time instead of separately. This will also lessen the duration of the discomfort.

With some painful procedures a topical anesthetic may be used to decrease the transmission of noxious stimuli, and the nurse should request such of the physician. Topical anesthetics cannot be absorbed through unbroken skin, but some effectively produce local anesthesia when they come in contact with mucous membranes or open wounds. For example, a topical anesthetic may be applied to an ulceration on the leg or to a nasogastric tube.

The patient whose diet is not restricted in any way may experience occasional minor discomfort because of improper food choices. Such a patient probably needs general diet counseling, but certain foods or diet changes may provide rapid or temporary relief. A slight burning sensation in the stomach may be quickly relieved by drinking milk. A patient with intestinal cramping associated with diarrhea may experience relief within hours if he decreases the amount of coffee he consumes, eats smaller amounts of food more frequently, and chooses foods low in residue. The abdominal discomfort and headache related to constipation may be relieved by a glass of prune juice. Or a warm lemonade may be made with hot water, the juice of half a lemon and two teaspoons of honey. The patient with slight burning on urination may find that the discomfort decreases when he drinks larger amounts of water.

One source of noxious stimuli postoperatively is thought to be reflexive spasms of muscles that have been divided or cut. A recent study indicates that moist heat is effective in reducing muscle spasm. With the physician's permission and written order, patients with abdominal surgery received hydrocollator packs to the wound for fifteen minutes, three times a day and as desired for the first four postoperative days. This reduced the number of narcotic analgesics required. The packs contain a silicone gel substance inside a canvas cover. When the packs are submerged in 170° F. water bath, they retain heat and moisture for about 30 minutes after they are removed. The pack is then placed in a terry cloth cover and positioned over the wound. The dressings become perceptibly moist, but cultures have revealed no problem with possible infection. These packs are rather heavy and this may be a source of discomfort to the patient. If the pack is too heavy or if a hydrocollator is not available, cotton or wool may be steamed or wrung from hot water and used in the same manner as the hydrocollator. This use of cotton or wool is less convenient since heat is not retained as long and the procedure of steaming or wringing must be repeated (Halsell).

Utilizing other professional assistance. The nurses and the physician giving care to a patient with pain may find that their skills are not providing the desired level of pain relief for the patient. Other specialists—physical therapists, occupational therapists, inhalation therapists, pharmacists, dietitians, radiologists and others—may be called upon in certain situations. In this section we will discuss some of the contributions of only four professional groups: social workers, clergymen, anesthesiologists and psychiatrists. And, a brief comment will be made about the use of hypnosis.

Generally speaking, the four professional groups listed above function in one or more of three interrelated areas. First, they may assist with the management of the cause of the pain. The anesthesiologist may be helpful with pain that originates with a physical stimulus. A psychiatrist may deal with emotional conflicts that result in a pain sensation. Secondly, they may assist with pain relief measures by managing some of the factors that increase the perceived intensity of pain or decrease pain tolerance. The clergyman, social worker or psychiatrist may contribute in this way. They may also contribute in a third way by assisting the patient to handle pain in a manner that minimizes the disruption to his total life style.

The social worker. The social worker may be an invaluable aid to the care of the patient with pain. Anxiety reduction is one of the common methods by which certain measures bring about pain relief. If anxiety remains high for any reason, pain relief may not be achieved. Although some of the factors responsible for high anxiety may be handled by the nurse, others require the assistance of a social worker. The social worker may help the patient and his family with financial problems resulting from illness. She may provide emotional support for the patient and his family before, during and after hospitalization. She may help family members cope with their concerns about the patient's condition. The social worker may be able to obtain housing close to the hospital for a family member such as a spouse who lives a great distance from the hospital but wishes to visit the patient daily. Because of the social worker's knowledge of community resources she may be able to obtain a variety of services for the patient and his family. The social worker may also be able to provide important information about the values, strengths and weaknesses of the patient's family. This information assists the nurse to be more realistic about ways in which family members can help the patient and more practical about plans for caring for the patient at home. Thus, by relieving the patient of some of his worries, and the family of theirs, she reduces mutual tension. The patient as a result probably will perceive less pain and tolerate it better.

Some of the social worker's contributions are illustrated in the case of Mr. Blair, 42 years old, in the third week of his hospitalization for metastatic carcinoma. A colostomy had been performed eighteen days previously, and Mr. Blair was receiving radiation therapy. He had been ill and unable to work for about four months, but the malignancy had not been discovered until the beginning of this hospitalization. Mr. Blair was generally in the middle socioeconomic status. He was employed as an engineer and lived in a modest suburban home with his wife and three children. He had two sons, four and seven years old, and one daughter, nine years old.

Mr. Blair was not expressive about his pain, but he appeared to be experiencing considerable discomfort almost constantly. Frequently, he lay motionless in bed, clenching his fists and perspiring. He requested his narcotic analgesic every three hours, and he often employed several of the pain relief measures the nurse had taught him. These included relaxation, rhythmic breathing and distraction. None, including the analgesics, seemed to be very effective. Upon questioning, Mr. Blair usually said his pain was only slightly less intense. Mr. Blair knew that his illness was serious; but since he had not asked about his prognosis, he had not been told that his life expectancy was six months to a year. However, his wife knew the illness was terminal. Mr. Blair seemed to handle his feelings about his illness by intellectualizing. The nurse helped him utilize this defense by providing and discussing such facts as the actions of certain medications and the care of his colostomy.

But Mr. Blair's inability to obtain a significant amount of pain relief indicated that there were other sources of anxiety besides the illness *per se*. The nurse discovered through her interactions with Mr. Blair that he was very concerned about the welfare of his family. She also observed that Mrs. Blair's anxiety was contributing to her husband's unrest. In addition to trying to cope with his impending death, Mrs. Blair had to handle some very practical and difficult problems of which her husband was also aware. Financial problems were becoming quite serious. Considering the previous and future medical bills, Mrs. Blair calculated she would either have to move to less expensive quarters or have no money for groceries. Their car could not be driven because it needed expensive repairs. Mrs. Blair had to travel twenty miles by bus to visit her husband. Since they had only recently moved to the area, they had no friends or relatives who could take care of the children while Mrs. Blair was at the hospital. She could not afford a babysitter for the four-year-old son, so she had to bring him with her on the bus. The child waited in the lobby because children were not allowed on the hospital units, and Mrs. Blair had to be checking on him constantly. She had to return home before her other children got out of school. In addition to these problems Mrs. Blair expressed to the nurse that she was worried about her children. She knew they were concerned about their father, but she did not have the energy to offer them much emotional support.

The nurse felt that if some of the family problems related to money, child care and transportation could be handled, Mr. Blair would experience less anxiety and obtain greater pain relief. In addition, Mrs. Blair would be less anxious and physically exhausted, and would have more energy to handle her husband's fatal illness and to offer him emotional support. The nurse then asked the social worker assigned to that hospital unit to see Mr. and Mrs. Blair. The social worker talked with the couple together and separately, and visited their home to determine the needs of the children. Through her knowledge of community resources the social worker obtained funds to have the car repaired. While this was being done she enlisted a volunteer to drive Mrs. Blair to and from the hospital. She told Mrs. Blair of a day care center where she could place the four-year-old for a nominal fee. The social worker contacted youth groups and young adult groups in the community. Certain members regularly saw the school-age children and provided them with entertainment, recreation, meals and an opportunity to work through their feelings about their disrupted home life and their father's illness. The social worker suggested to Mrs. Blair that she find out from her husband what insurance policies they had and where he kept copies and records of insurance. The social worker then assisted Mrs. Blair to understand the benefits of the insurance and to make the appropriate medical claims. With the money obtained through the insurance plus contributions from some community groups, the social worker helped Mrs. Blair devise a budget that would not require her to move to a less expensive home. The social worker continued to work with the family and showed them how to obtain other types of assistance. Both the social worker and the nurse frequently talked with Mrs. Blair to help her through the grief and mourning process.

Within a few days after the social worker's initial contact, Mrs. Blair was much more calm and supportive in the presence of her husband. Mr. Blair expressed confidence in the social worker and said to the nurse, "I'm sure glad you called in a social worker. She knows what she's doing, and she's going to help us see this thing through. There are a lot of things I could take care of if I didn't feel so bad. She's really helped my wife." One of Mr. Blair's most frequent comments related to his lawn; prior to his illness he had taken great pride in its care. The social worker had found a young boy to volunteer to mow and water the lawn. Often and with great satisfaction Mr. Blair would say, "It's really good to know that someone's taking care of my yard." Conversation about his lawn became a distraction from his pain, whereas before it had been a source of sadness.

Through the social worker's efforts Mr. Blair received more support from his wife and was less worried about his family and home. In essence the social worker assisted with the management of factors that had increased the patient's anxiety and consequently had decreased his ability to deal with pain. She also was able to minimize the effect the patient's illness and pain had on his life style and that of his family. This seemed to increase the effectiveness of pain relief measures, since

Mr. Blair began to experience some periods of almost complete pain relief.

The clergyman. For the patient who is committed to and practices a religious belief, a clergyman of that faith may make many contributions to the enhancement of pain relief. The clergyman may visit the patient at home or in the hospital, and he may ask members of the church to visit. Church groups often aid the patient and his family by providing food, money, transportation, babysitting, clothing and housekeeping. These services may result indirectly in pain relief because they enable family members to be with the patient and because they reduce the patient's concern about his home and family. Also, the patient may derive pain relief from the distraction of visits from church members.

The clergyman himself may enable the patient to find ways of coping with pain. Many patients look to their religions for answers and understanding regarding illness and pain. The clergyman may help the patient with this and assist him to find strength and inner peace through prayer. The clergyman may alleviate some of the anxiety, guilt, depression or loneliness associated with pain by emphasizing that God's love and spirit are with the patient throughout his pain. By talking, reading scriptures and praying with the patient, the clergyman may help the patient become relaxed and tranquil. In a variety of ways the clergyman may assist the patient to utilize the resources of his religious faith. If the patient in pain professes to be religious, the nurse should suggest that he contact his clergyman, or she may ask a clergyman associated with the hospital to visit the patient. She may also ask the patient if he wishes to have religious literature or symbols at his bedside.

Occasionally a patient in pain is particularly upset because he has misinterpreted the teachings of his religion. The patient may be angry with God because he believes God has caused his pain. Or, he may fear that his pain is God's way of punishing him for a sin. This may be a devastating experience for the patient who has previously been comforted by prayer. If he is angry with God, or feels that God is punishing him, he may no longer be comforted by his faith and may be less able to tolerate pain. This situation occurred in the case of Mrs. Carver, a patient with sudden and severe pain. Her level of arousal had been lowered by analgesics and other drugs, and this seemed to prevent her from reconciling her pain with her religious beliefs. Mrs. Carver moaned and tossed and turned in bed, crying out, "How could You desert me, God? Why have You let this happen to me? What have I done to deserve this?" The nurse knew that Mrs. Carver had found strength in prayer during her illness. She realized that Mrs. Carver needed religious guidance at that point, and called the clergyman affiliated with the hospital. He arrived at once, took Mrs. Carver's hand,

and began talking with her. Soon he began praying, and the nurse heard him say, "God, in our hour of pain help us remember Your love. Help us know that You are with us always. Our lives on earth are plagued with problems that You do not cause, but You help us through them. Help us understand that You are a kind and loving God, always forgiving and ready to help us even if we fail You. Help us know that You do not inflict pain to punish us but that we punish ourselves by not turning to You for strength." At the end of this prayer Mrs. Carver was lying relaxed in bed, looking at the clergyman with dazed eyes. In an effort to relate to Mrs. Carver in terms of her lowered cognitive ability, the clergyman then said, "Repeat after me: God loves me. God is with me." Mrs. Carver closed her eyes and repeated the words several times. As a result, Mrs. Carver's anxiety was decreased and she began to relax. After the clergyman left, Mrs. Carver said, "I feel better now. I can stand it." The relaxation and anxiety reduction that resulted when her faith in God was restored contributed to pain relief in several ways. It seemed to enable her to perceive a decreased intensity of pain, to tolerate the remaining pain, and to benefit from other pain relief measures.

The anesthesiologist. The anesthesiologist has almost daily experiences with a number of drugs and procedures that may be used to provide pain relief for patients other than those undergoing operative procedures. He employs general anesthetics, regional and local anesthetics, analgesics, sedatives and muscle relaxants. He is especially skilled in performing local and regional nerve blocks and has considerable experience with the recognition and treatment of complications arising from these procedures.

The physician responsible for the patient's care is usually the health team member who recognizes the need for consultation with an anesthesiologist. Because of the anesthesiologist's special skills, the physician often requests that he perform a nerve block procedure when it is indicated. However, the nurse may suggest to the physician that an anesthesiologist be consulted. Most often the services of the anesthesiologist are indicated when the patient experiences severe and uncontrollable pain, especially if it is chronic. The anesthesiologist may administer a regional or local anesthetic. Depending upon the agent selected, a nerve block may be permanent or it may last only a few hours. The following are examples of procedures the anesthesiologist may use to control pain. (Some may also be helpful in diagnosing the cause of pain or in determining the effectiveness of a neurosurgical procedure for pain relief.) Spinal blocks may be used for the relief of intractable pain of carcinoma in the abdomen, pelvis or lower extremities. An epidural block may relieve the pain of vasospastic disease or arterial occlusion in the lower body and may improve peripheral circulation. A stellate ganglion block may provide pain relief in Raynaud's disease or malignancy of the neck. A muscle spasm may be relieved by infiltrating it with a local anesthetic (Eckenhoff). Knowing that these are the types of pain relief methods most anesthesiologists are able to administer, the nurse will have some idea of when consultation with an anesthesiologist may be beneficial.

The psychiatrist. A psychiatrist may contribute to the treatment of pain in any one of the three ways mentioned at the beginning of this section. He may assist the patient and/or the patient's family (1) to deal with emotional conflicts that result in a pain sensation, (2) to manage factors that increase anxiety or depression and thereby increase pain, and (3) to minimize disruption in life style. Thus, the psychiatrist may assist the patient with pain either by treating the cause of the pain or by assisting the patient toward better methods of coping with it. A clinical psychologist may also make these contributions, but the psychiatrist's medical background puts him in a somewhat better position to work with the patient in pain.

The physician caring for the patient with pain is usually the person who makes a referral to the psychiatrist or requests a consultation with him. However, the nurse should be able to recognize some of the circumstances that indicate the possible need for a psychiatrist. The nurse may suggest a psychiatric consultation if the physician is fairly sure that the patient's pain originates with or is sustained by emotional conflicts; if the patient's pain, regardless of its cause, is persistent or severe and seems to be increased by affects such as anxiety or depression; or if the patient's life style is disrupted considerably because of his pain or the affects resulting from the pain. In other words, the psychiatrist is a valuable resource when pain relief seems to be dependent upon achieving structural changes in the patient's personality, providing intensive emotional support to the patient and/or his family, or assisting the patient to find ways of coping with pain that lessen the extent of changes that must be made in his life style.

Some of the psychiatrist's contributions to the management of pain and one nursing approach to helping the patient accept psychiatric help will be illustrated briefly in the case of Mr. Bonner. Mr. Bonner, 52 years old, was admitted for treatment of an acute attack of gout. Gout had been diagnosed for a year. Mr. Bonner had continued working although he stated that he constantly felt pain. His wife of 23 years said he had tolerated the pain well but had become progressively more irritable during the last few months. She added that he was very discouraged about his current acute attack of severe pain. During this hospitalization it became evident that Mr. Bonner's energy for coping with pain had been exhausted. His wife and physician were surprised that this usually rather mild-mannered man with a good sense of humor suddenly had episodes of extreme anger, which alternated with periods of refusing to talk to anyone and failing to comply with treatments. He would usually respond to efforts to explore with him the meaning of his pain, but these conversations resulted in little if any pain relief or behavior change. Some of his comments were: "I can't face thinking about years and years of even a little bit of pain every day." "This pain is bad, but that nagging pain has destroyed my life." On two occasions the physician told Mr. Bonner that he could probably go home the next day. Discharge from the hospital was delayed both times because Mr. Bonner began complaining of pain too severe to allow him to go home. It seemed possible that going home meant to him that he would be confronted once again with unacceptable changes in his way of living. The anxiety and depression associated with this disruption seemed to increase the duration and severity of his pain. Mr. Bonner also needed help in re-establishing his former coping style and perhaps in finding new coping strategies. Therefore, the nurse discussed this with his physician and suggested the aid of a psychiatrist. The physician agreed to talk with the patient about this possibility.

After the physician had asked Mr. Bonner to think about discussing his feelings with a psychiatrist, the nurse talked with Mr. Bonner. Mr. Bonner opened the conversation with, "I guess they think I'm crazy. My doctor wants me to see a psychiatrist. That doctor's crazy himself if he thinks this pain is all in my head." This is typical of a patient's reaction to the suggestion of seeing a psychiatrist about pain. The patient often thinks that a psychiatrist only treats "crazy people" or "imaginary pain." Frequently the use of a psychiatrist must be approached cautiously with the patient, allowing ample time for the patient to understand what is being advocated and why. The nurse replied to Mr. Bonner, "No one thinks you're crazy. People often talk with psychiatrists when they're having especially difficult problems. Everyone knows that living with pain day after day is very hard." Mr. Bonner agreed, but wanted to know what the psychiatrist could do about his pain. The nurse explained, "A psychiatrist helps people find ways to help themselves. The psychiatrist will probably talk with you about how this discomfort makes you feel. For example, doesn't the discomfort upset you a lot sometimes? And, doesn't this make you even more uncomfortable?" Mr. Bonner thought this was true and elaborated on the relationship between his emotions and his pain. The nurse talked with Mr. Bonner once more that day. At the end of the conversation she suggested that Mr. Bonner ask the psychiatrist to drop by so that he could find out more about what a psychiatrist might have to offer him. Mr. Bonner said he would do this, and the psychiatrist saw him the next day.

The psychiatrist felt that Mr. Bonner would benefit from a short period of therapy. By the end of the week Mr. Bonner had seen the psychiatrist three more times, and was able to leave the hospital. Three months after his discharge the nurse made a point of finding out when Mr. Bonner had his next appointment in the medical outpatient clinic. The nurse saw him during that appointment, and Mr. Bonner commented. "I'm still seeing that psychiatrist. He's helped me some. I'm able to keep working. I didn't realize how angry I was about this pain. He helps me see when I'm getting angry and I can do something about it. It's not easy to live this way, but I'll manage." Mr. Bonner saw the psychiatrist weekly for six months. The psychiatrist reported to the nurse that Mr. Bonner eventually was able to cope successfully with his daily discomfort. By suggesting a psychiatrist to Mr. Bonner's physician and by assisting Mr. Bonner to accept the help of the psychiatrist, the nurse contributed to Mr. Bonner's ability to live with his pain with less disruption in his manner of living.

The psychiatrist may be asked to assist with the diagnosis and treatment of the patient with pain originating with or sustained by emotional conflicts. Phantom pain is one example of pain the psychiatrist may be asked to treat. Sternbach's (1968) review of the literature suggests that neurosurgical procedures are distressingly unsuccessful in relieving phantom pain. He feels that patients so afflicted need the pain to deal with an underlying but not overt depression. Psychotherapy and electroshock therapy have been frequently successful in achieving pain relief. With some patients no specific label seems to apply, yet emotional conflicts appear to be related to the disease process or the occurrence of pain.

It is often difficult to determine the extent to which the patient's emotional conflicts contribute to pain. Pain that originates with or is sustained by emotional conflicts cannot be identified by any particular qualities or characteristics. Sometimes the patient's pain is of brief duration, but more often it has existed for months or years. The pain may be located in any one or several areas of the body. It may take the form of phantom limb pain, abdominal pain, "pain all over," backaches or headaches. The intensity may range from mild to severe, remain the same, or fluctuate. The presence of cellular changes does not rule out the possibility that the pain had originally been psychogenic. And, of course, cellular changes occur in the organ neuroses. Psychogenic pain may eventually evoke peripheral, reflexive changes that resemble the processes of a physical disease, and these changes may be sufficient to account for the pain. Similarly, the inability to detect organic processes capable of producing pain is no guarantee that such organic processes do not exist. Diagnostic tools may not be sensitive enough to reveal the organic processes. Further, the presence of emotional problems does not automatically mean that the patient's pain is psychogenic or even an organ neurosis. The patient suffering from pain of physical origin very often develops anxiety, depression or preoccupation with the pain. However, from the physician's point of view it is necessary to make a differential diagnosis because the physician must find and treat the threatening physical illness before it is too late to alter the course of the disease. He must also recognize the extent to which the patient's psychological makeup contributes to the illness if he is to rehabilitate the patient (Alexander).

It should be pointed out that the nurse's role in the care of the patient with psychogenic pain or an organ neurosis does not differ basically from her care of any other patient with pain. The processes of nursing assessment, intervention and evaluation remain the same unless the physician or psychiatrist suggests otherwise. There are, however, at least three things that may require more of the nurse's attention than usual.

First, the nurse may find it difficult to help the patient accept psychiatric help. As the example of Mr. Bonner illustrates, the patient is likely to fear that the suggestion of a psychiatrist means that others do not really believe he feels pain. The nurse must take special care to convey to the patient that she does believe he feels a sensation of pain. The patient, like Mr. Bonner, may also fail to understand how a psychiatrist can help him. It has been suggested that the time to introduce the idea of seeing a psychiatrist is when the patient himself relates his pain to his other problems (Tingling and Klein).

Secondly, more of the nurse's attention may be directed toward preventing or controlling situations that tend to precipitate emotional conflicts in the patient. For example, if the patient becomes very upset if his wife does not visit him daily, the nurse may help the wife make arrangements to do so. Or, the nurse may spend more time with the patient when his wife does not visit.

Thirdly, the nurse may have difficulty handling her own feelings when she cares for the patient. In a sense, the patient needs his pain and uses it to deal with emotional problems. It is not always easy for the nurse to accept the patient's inability to cope with his emotions in some other way. Perhaps the most difficult part of caring for this type of patient is that he does not respond well to pain relief measures. This may be very discouraging to the nurse, and she may be tempted to cease her efforts to help the patient. These feelings are not restricted to the nurse. Physicians also tend to be angered and frustrated with such a patient. Often the patient is sent from one physician to another. The nurse should recognize that her feelings of failure or her anger toward the patient are not unusual. In addition to trying to gain a better understanding of the patient's situation, she may need to be relieved of his care for a few days.

Once the patient agrees to a consultation with the psychiatrist, the nurse should not expect a miracle. A long period of psychotherapy may be indicated, the expected results may be quite limited, and the patient's progress may be slow. The psychiatrist may decide that therapy is not indicated even though emotional conflicts are basic to the patient's pain. Sometimes the psychiatrist feels that he can do nothing for the patient, but that continued medical supervision is necessary. Or, he may feel that suffering would be greater if the patient were to relinquish the pain and try to deal with his emotional problems. One psychiatrist makes a compassionate plea for recognizing and accepting those patients in whom relief of pain would be more devastating than the persistence of pain (Szasz).

Hypnosis. Regardless of the cause of the patient's pain, whether it originates with a physical or emotional stimulus, hypnosis may be considered as a technique for providing pain relief. Hypnosis is not likely to be effective with the depressed patient, since it appears to produce pain relief through anxiety reduction. Psychogenic pain is often associated with an underlying but not overt depression. Therefore, hypnosis may be less effective with these types of patients.

Although hypnosis has been used for hundreds of years, it is not yet completely understood. However, the nurse should realize that hypnosis is a legitimate and sometimes very effective form of treatment when it is used in the proper circumstances. In 1958 the American Medical Association accepted hypnosis as a therapeutic technique but advised caution. The use of hypnosis is not limited to any one professional or non-professional group. Anyone of average intelligence may learn the hypnotic technique within a few hours. But hypnosis should be used only under the supervision of a physician. The use of hypnosis by amateurs may unwittingly precipitate an emotional disturbance in a few subjects.

When hypnosis is used for the purpose of pain relief, the results will depend upon the patient's susceptibility to suggestion and the nature of the suggestions made. The patient may experience anesthesia, or insensitivity, of the painful area. Or, analgesia may result, ranging from a decrease in the perceived intensity of pain to a state of not caring about the pain. Even if the patient is not very susceptible to suggestions, hypnosis often produces relaxation.

Aside from the mystique surrounding hypnotism, there are other more realistic reasons for the limited use of this technique in the treatment of pain. Hypnotic anesthesia or analgesia can be produced in only a small percentage of the population. And, the use of hypnosis requires a great deal of the patient's and hypnotist's time and effort. Many sessions over a period of days or months may be necessary, and the patient may be required to practice self-hypnosis between sessions.

Being with the patient. Here we are concerned with the simple presence of the nurse—being with the patient without necessarily saying or doing anything. In Sternbach's (1968) words "we are never quite so alone as when we are in pain" (p. 84). The presence of the nurse may not always eliminate the patient's feeling of isolation but it may reduce it. Because pain crowds out other stimuli, the patient may continue to feel alone although the nurse is with him. On the other hand, when the patient is aware that the nurse is with him his loneliness, anxiety or other affects associated with pain may be alleviated. This will contribute to pain relief. At other times the presence of the nurse may only prevent an increase in the pain and anxiety.

There are several situations in which simply being with the patient may be the single most appropriate nursing activity for pain relief or control. These primarily include those times when the patient is too fatigued to talk with anyone, when the patient is completely occupied with some other pain-relief activity such as the Lamaze method or waking-imagined analgesia, when all possible pain relief measures have been applied and the patient has not responded, and when the patient cannot talk and will not accept touch. The latter may occur with the child who is crying and trying to escape from the adults he fears. Or the fatigued adult male may not be comfortable with the dependency inherent in touch.

Some of the situations in which simply being with the adult is important are also circumstances in which the nurse may find it difficult to be with the patient. Many nurses are much more comfortable if they are doing something with their hands or at least talking with the patient. In addition, the difficulty of being with the patient is increased when the patient responds to pain in a manner not prescribed by the nurse's culture. If the nurse is from the Old American culture she may be embarrassed when an adult male patient moans, cries or screams in response to pain. This type of patient is all too frequently left alone with his pain. The nurse's understanding of cultural influences, as discussed in Chapter 3, may assist her to remain with this patient. If she leaves him he may feel that he has alienated her and other staff members, and he may fear he has been deserted. Many times the patient is aware that his responses to pain are unacceptable in the cultural group to which the staff belong. But, it is extremely difficult for him to change his responses. He may also feel it is unnatural to act in another way.

There is another problem perhaps more significant than the nurse's difficulty with being inactive or accepting responses to pain that differ from hers. It is the problem of coping with the fact that some pain is inevitable and she may not be able to do much about it. In this respect both the nurse and the patient have to endure the pain. Both may feel helpless, and the nurse in particular may feel failure acutely. Sometimes the nurse's efforts not only fail to contribute to pain relief but inadvertently she may have caused more pain through some theoretically sound measure such as repositioning. The situation becomes even more difficult for the nurse to witness when the patient becomes angry or blames the nurse as the child is likely to do.

It is natural to want to escape these signs of failure. How does the nurse handle her sense of failure so that she is able to remain with the patient? Whether or not the patient hears or understands, it sometimes helps the nurse to say, "I'm sorry. I've done all I can and now I'll just stay here with you if you want." Other times the nurse must leave the room to regain her composure. If possible, it is advantageous to discuss the situation with someone else. In any event, the nurse can recall what she has done for the patient, be sure that she has not overlooked any other possibilities for pain relief, and realize that the pain may be unavoidable. Then she may consider that her only realistic failure may be that of abandoning the patient.

The effectiveness of simply being with the patient is exemplified by a situation involving a nurse and Mr. Harris. Mr. Harris was admitted to a private room from the emergency unit with a pneumothorax and other injuries sustained in an automobile accident. Closed-chest drainage had been established. He had received only a small dose of morphine because of the danger of depressing respirations. Through questioning and observation the nurse ascertained that in addition to a continuous and moderate degree of chest pain he also felt intense, intermittent abdominal pain of undetermined origin. He manifested this intense pain by wrinkling of the brow, increase in pulse rate, and a soft moan. Initially, Mr. Harris' participation in structured and purposeful distraction effectively decreased the intensity of the intermittent abdominal pains. Eventually fatigue, previous loss of blood and many other factors combined to lower his level of consciousness. He no longer was able to utilize distraction, and further medication was contraindicated. He began dozing, waking up with manifestations of the intense abdominal pain. At this time the nurse left the room to report the patient's condition to the physician. She returned ten minutes later to find Mr. Harris moaning much louder and clutching the sheets. There were no indications of a change in his medical status, and he nodded affirmatively when the nurse asked if this were the same abdominal pain. When he seemed to doze again the nurse started to leave the room. Mr. Harris opened his eyes and asked, "Are you leaving?" The nurse replied, "I'll be glad to stay if you want me to." Mr. Harris replied, "Please," and began to doze again. The nurse sat beside his bed. From time to time he opened his eyes, glanced around the room, and closed his eyes again after he saw the nurse. When he experienced abdominal pain he would look for the nurse and manifest his pain as he had initially. There were no more incidents of loud moaning and clutching the sheets. The patient's awareness of the nurse's presence apparently decreased his anxiety and consequently decreased the perceived intensity of pain.

When the nurse's other responsibilities prevent her from remaining with the patient, frequent, regular, brief visits can be substituted. For example, the nurse could have assured Mr. Harris that she would come to his bedside every five to ten minutes. When she came she could have waited for him to see her before leaving again. The nurse's regular visits can be combined with securing an agency volunteer or a member of the patient's family to remain with the patient. Of course, some patients will prefer that an "expert" such as the nurse be present, but realistically this is not always possible.

Being with the patient is especially important during the latter stages of the anticipation of pain. Anxiety tends to increase as the time approaches to engage in a painful event. The desire to be with another person usually increases as anxiety increases (Schachter). The nurse's presence may reduce the anticipatory anxiety and thereby reduce the amount of anxiety present when the pain sensation occurs. This may lessen the perceived intensity of the pain. Remaining with the patient also allows him the opportunity to initiate an interaction when he desires it and feels able to do so. At some point the patient may be able to use the nurse as a form of distraction, discuss his feelings with her, or simply reach out for her hand.

As effective as the nurse's presence may be for some patients in certain circumstances, she must be alert to those patients who would rather be alone or be with someone else such as a family member. In the discussion of cultural influence mention was made of patients who want to be alone when their pain becomes intense. For example, the Old American places value on minimal responses to pain. When pain becomes intense he may prefer to be alone for fear he will lose control of his behavior. The Irishman does not mind admitting he has pain but prefers to suffer alone. He has some pride in being able to handle his pain through either relaxing or fighting, but he seems to need to be alone to use these techniques. The preference for being alone with pain may, therefore, be based on different reasons for different patients. And, of course, the desire to be alone with pain is not limited to membership in a particular cultural group. In addition, the patient may want the nurse to be absent if a procedure involves a socially unacceptable body part. For example, a male patient may prefer that a female nurse leave if he is being catheterized for urine retention.

The desire to be with a family member or friend other than the nurse may occur in the case of a child or an adult. The young child in particular may feel safer and less anxious about pain if he is with his mother rather than the nurse. Or, when a husband and wife have practiced the Lamaze method together, the prospective mother may feel much more confident and less anxious during labor if her husband is allowed to remain with her.

The effectiveness of the presence of a family member rather than the nurse is demonstrated by Mrs. Billings at the beginning of her third hospitalization for incision and drainage of recurrent, multiple breast abscesses. No anesthetics were used since the patient was sensitive to local anesthetics and the frequency of incision and drainage precluded the use of a general anesthetic. Prior to this particular incision and drainage Mrs. Billings said to the nurse, "It really isn't that bad. I've had it done so many times before. It's just that this time seems to bother me more and I really don't know why." After the patient refused the nurse's offer to stay during the procedure, the nurse began to explore the patient's comment by asking her to describe the last time the procedure was done. The patient remarked that her husband had been with her, but would not be present this time. The nurse asked Mrs. Billings if she thought it would help to have her husband there and if it would be possible for him to arrive in time for the procedure. The patient immediately called her husband and he arrived in time. When the nurse came to administer Demerol, the patient refused the injection, saying "I don't need it. I'll be just fine now." This illustrates how the presence of someone other than the nurse can contribute to pain relief by reducing anxiety.

What are some nursing activities that can be used during the aftermath of pain?

The aftermath of pain, the third phase of the patient's pain experience, occurs when pain ceases or is substantially reduced. This period immediately following the presence of pain is a relatively neglected area of nursing intervention. When health team members believe that the pain is over or under control, they usually turn their attention elsewhere. However, the patient does not always realize that the pain is actually under control and may anticipate more to come. Further, the patient does not immediately forget about his pain, especially if it has been severe or frightening. At times the patient's reaction following the occurrence of pain sensations is somewhat similar to what most of us have experienced or witnessed following a life-threatening event. We may calmly and efficiently perform emergency external cardiac massage or skillfully maneuver an automobile to avoid an accident, but afterwards we may suddenly begin shaking and feeling faint and clammy. In the aftermath phase of pain these feelings as well as nausea, vomiting, chills and nightmares about the pain have been reported by patients.

Clearly, the patient needs some type of assistance during the aftermath phase of the pain experience. If it is likely that pain will recur, the nurse should employ pain relief measures previously suggested in this chapter. But once the pain is controlled and regardless of whether or not it may recur, there are at least two types of nursing intervention that are specific to the aftermath phase of pain and should be employed at that time. First, the nurse may need to inform the patient that the cause of pain has been removed or decreased. Secondly, the nurse may need to assist the patient with assimilation of the painful experience (McCaffery and Moss).

Conveying that the source of noxious stimuli has been removed or decreased. This nursing activity should not be confused with telling the patient that he no longer feels pain. The patient is the only judge of that. But the nurse may inform him that something has been done to diminish the cause of his pain. Sometimes pain is intermittent, and during pain-free periods the patient anticipates more pain. If the patient does not know that the cause of the pain has been removed or decreased, he probably will continue to anticipate pain and his anxiety may remain needlessly high. In his anxiety he may interpret as painful such sensations as touch and cold.

Diagnostic or therapeutic procedures such as a spinal tap or a thoracentesis are common types of situations in which the patient needs to be informed that the cause of pain has ceased or diminished. During a procedure the patient may experience intermittent discomfort of various types such as pressure or pricking. If he does not understand what the procedure involves or if he cannot see the procedure being done, he may not know when certain painful aspects are over. Once the procedure itself is completed, the patient often remains in the same position while health team members cleanse and bandage him and clear away the equipment. Thus, unless someone tells him what is happening, he receives no clues suggesting he need not anticipate further pain. For example, while the physician was cleansing the skin following a bone marrow aspiration of the ilium, the nurse noted that the patient continued with the same behavior he had manifested during the procedure. The muscles in his extremities remained tense, and he had not stopped using distraction for pain relief. He was looking at the ceiling and giving a detailed description of his stamp collection. The nurse said to the patient, "Mr. Henry, the doctor is finished with the bone marrow. He's just wiping your skin now." Mr. Henry relaxed immediately and began talking with the physician. By telling the patient that the noxious stimuli had ceased, the nurse prevented further manifestations of anxiety and anticipation of pain.

With the young child, verbal information will not necessarily be effective in conveying that no more noxious stimuli will be inflicted. For instance, following an injection the infant or toddler may continue to cry. To help him to understand that there will be no more injections at that time and to tolerate the residual discomfort, the nurse may change his position or pick him up and cuddle him. If a toddler or somewhat older child undergoes a painful procedure in a treatment room, he may not cease to anticipate pain until he is taken from the room. Efforts to distract the child and focus his attention on some pleasant stimulus such as a toy or eating is another method of conveying that the cause of pain has ceased or decreased.

The nurse must be careful not to convey that the cause of pain will cease completely if this is not likely to be the case. The nurse should avoid announcing prematurely that a procedure has been completed. For example, once the needle has entered the skin for a venipuncture, the nurse should not say the procedure is over. Further discomfort may occur from probing to find the vein or doing another puncture if the vein is not entered.

In other situations the nurse may inadvertently cause the patient to expect discomfort to disappear. This occurred with Mrs. Ellison who was in labor and was using the Lamaze method of childbirth. The following account is summarized from Mrs. Ellison's written narrative of her labor and delivery which she submitted to her Lamaze instructor. (Teachers of the Lamaze method often request this type of information so that they can evaluate their teaching and the effectiveness of the Lamaze method). Mrs. Ellison did not request or receive analgesics or anesthetics during her labor. Although she stated the pain was severe, she remained relaxed throughout labor and never cried or screamed with the contractions. On the way to the delivery room the physician told Mrs. Ellison she was going to receive a local anesthetic for the delivery. The nurse added, "It will be all over in a few minutes." A few more contractions occurred before the anesthetic was administered. Then, between contractions, Mrs. Ellison was told that the local anesthetic had been done. With the next contraction the patient began screaming loudly and saying, "I can feel it. It's hurting. I can feel it." Mrs. Ellison explained in her report, "When I heard I was going to get that anesthetic, I guess I wasn't thinking clearly. The nurse said *it* would be all over. I thought she meant the pain would go away when the local was done. So I prepared myself for only two or three more contractions. After I knew the local had been done, I thought that was it. When I felt more pain I just couldn't take it. It was too late to start my breathing (Lamaze rhythmic breathing pattern). I know I screamed awfully loud. I was just out of control." It is not unusual for a fatigued patient experiencing severe pain to misunderstand what is said. Because of a misunderstanding Mrs. Ellison failed to employ measures that had assisted her to tolerate the pain, and she experienced the embarrassment of losing control. This patient also exemplifies what may happen when a person prepares himself to tolerate a certain amount of pain. When pain occurs beyond what the patient expects, he may panic and perceive a greater intensity of pain or be unable to tolerate it. Misinterpretation of what the nurse said might have been prevented if the nurse had said that the baby would be born soon and not that "it" would be over. The nurse might also have explained to Mrs. Ellison that she would continue to feel the contractions.

Assisting with assimilation of the painful experience. People often talk about their painful experiences long after the pain sensations have ceased. Sometimes a person's story about pain seems to be a way of seeking praise and admiration for having endured it. In other cases the person seems to be trying to convince himself that the pain actually occurred; he is almost in awe of the painful experience. Still another person appears to be looking for answers and explanations about the pain or about himself; he does not seem to have a clear idea of all that happened or is not sure how to evaluate himself in terms of his responses to pain. The adult usually expresses these feelings verbally, but the child commonly reveals such feelings in a more dramatic and sometimes poignant manner. Reminders of almost all aspects of the child's illness, including pain, are frequently found in his bedside table. He may collect the cotton balls or syringe cases from each injection, the brightly colored Band Aids from venipunctures or finger pricks, or a gauze flat containing the sutures removed from his wound. The child often proudly displays these items in much the same way as an adult who has been awarded a medal or trophy for an outstanding per-formance in sports or some other venture. The child's small treasures seem to symbolize what he has accomplished: He has endured pain. His trophies help him celebrate and mark the end of pain. The reminders of his pain also seem to help him understand what has happened to him since they are tangible aspects of an otherwise elusive experience (McCaffery, 1969).

The behavior of Jason, a seven-year-old boy, illustrates how the child may use an item associated with pain to celebrate the cessation of pain and to express pride in being able to endure pain. After Jason's sutures and suprapubic catheter were removed, he twirled the catheter above his head, smiling and laughing. He excitedly shouted to the nurse at the other end of the ward, "They took it out. It's all over. I had an operation and I'm OK. No more hurts. It's all over." The nurse said very little to him because she was busy with a dressing change on another child, but Jason continued to twirl the catheter and talk for about twenty minutes. He reluctantly allowed the nurse to take away the catheter to wash it for him.

In the aftermath of pain not all children and adults are as joyous and expressive as Jason. It is not unusual for the patient to need assistance in assimilating an occurrence of pain. In other words, the patient may need help with the intellectual and emotional incorporation of a painful event. The process of assisting the patient to assimilate an occurrence of pain involves encouraging him to express what he remembers about the characteristics of the painful sensation, his emotions and thoughts during his pain, his overt responses to the pain, and what other people were doing and saying while it was happening. One of these aspects of his painful experience may be of more concern to him than others, but he may not realize how upsetting a certain aspect is until he begins to recall it.

In a way the nurse encourages the patient to reenact or relive the pain. The manner in which this is done depends upon the patient's cognitive ability. Most alert adults simply talk about the pain. However, if it was an especially frightening event that the patient cannot recall clearly, it may be helpful to reconstruct the situation by taking the patient to the room where the pain occurred and showing him some of the equipment associated with it. Of course, this should not be forced upon the patient who says he does not want to remember. These details may not be as important to him as his emotional feelings about the pain.

Because of the child's cognitive level, the process of assimilating pain is usually facilitated by a play situation. The painful event may be reconstructed by giving the child dolls that symbolize himself and the people involved with his pain. He should also be given the same or similar equipment used during the pain. The nurse may suggest that the child "play like" one of the dolls is having the same painful experience he had. With the nurse's assistance he can perform procedures on the doll.

A question often arises about the potential physical danger of giving the child the actual equipment associated with his pain, especially if it includes needles or other sharp instruments. If a child is old enough to understand that the equipment is dangerous and if he can handle objects with manual dexterity, there seems to be no reason why he cannot be allowed to manipulate sharp objects as long as the nurse supervises him and does not leave him alone with the equipment. This author has given a doll and a syringe with a needle attached to many young children to assist them with the assimilation of intramuscular injections. No accidents have ever occurred and no child ever deliberately tried to hurt himself or the nurse. The very hostile and angry child usually only stabs the doll vigorously and does not strike out at the nurse. Initially such a child may be afraid to touch the syringe and may be very hesitant about giving the doll an injection. But after a few more opportunities he often becomes quite expressive about his feelings.

During the process of assisting the child or adult to assimilate his pain, the nurse may discover that the patient has an inaccurate or incomplete understanding of the facts. This is especially likely to occur with the child. For example, following open heart surgery the child may believe that his heart has been removed, or following a tonsillectomy the young female child may be so totally confused as to believe that the physician has removed an unborn baby from her abdomen. The child is prone to develop fantasies of mutilation. Repeated sessions of doll play may correct these misconceptions and relieve anxiety. The child may begin to understand that, as bad as it was, he was not in a torture chamber surrounded by monsters. For instance, following a lumbar puncture which the child cannot see, play with a doll and needle may assist the child to understand that he was not cut with a knife or that the needle was not after all quite as big as he had thought.

In addition to providing information during the process of assisting the adult or child to assimilate pain, the nurse may also find that the patient needs praise or reassurance about his behavioral responses to pain. The child or adult may fear that others think he was a "sissy" about the pain. Or, the adult may be more concerned about his own concept of himself than he is about the opinions of others. He may have always thought of himself as capable of controlling his behavior in all situations. He may experience considerable anxiety if he feels he lost control during pain. To re-establish the patient's self-concept or to assure him that others do not disapprove of him, the nurse usually should tell the patient that he handled his pain well, regardless of how he behaved. Sometimes it helps the patient to know that other patients behave similarly during experiences such as his. If the patient values control and minimally expressive behavior, the nurse can usually find some part of the patient's behavior that was consistent with his values, focus on it and praise the patient for it. Besides verbal praise and reassurance, the child should be allowed to keep some souvenir or trophy, of his choice if possible. The child can display his "badge of courage" to others and obtain further approval. Since this award is often a symbol of reality, or of what really happened, it may also serve to minimize frightening fantasies. Adults, too, sometimes collect souvenirs of pain such as gallstones.

The effect of assisting the patient to assimilate his pain has not been studied sufficiently to know exactly what this accomplishes for the patient. The knowledge, praise and reassurance the patient gains as well as the opportunity to express his feelings often seem to have an immediate effect of dissipating anxiety. But when no efforts are made to help the patient assimilate pain, anxiety and other emotional feelings about the pain may linger long after the pain sensations have ceased.

This was demonstrated by Mrs. Ellison who was mentioned in the preceding section. Her narrative was written six weeks after her labor and delivery and included some of her feelings after the painful experience. She said that on the day she was discharged from the hospital she developed a spinal headache and some mild muscle spasms in her upper back. Her physician asked her if she wanted to take home any medication for the discomfort. She replied, "Oh, yes. I must have something. Since my labor I'm panicked about pain." A while later Mrs. Ellison told one of the nurses that she wanted to talk about her labor. The nurse sat down and listened for about ten minutes. They were interrupted and the conversation was never resumed. Mrs. Ellison's concern about her pain persisted after she went home. Her labor had begun on a Monday and ended on a Tuesday. She said that every Monday and Tuesday for the six weeks following childbirth, she recalled exactly what had happened during her labor. Every time she looked at a clock on those days she remembered, without wanting to, what had been going on and how she had felt at that time during her labor. During her fourth week postpartum she reported several nightmares about her labor and delivery. Interestingly enough, Mrs. Ellison was concerned as much about the labor she had tolerated without analgesics or anesthetics as she was about the delivery when she had screamed.

Mrs. Ellison's narrative clearly indicates that she needed assistance with assimilation of her pain. It also suggests that the patient who tolerates pain well may have as great a need to assimilate the experiece as the patient who seems to have considerable difficulty tolerating pain. Further, Mrs. Ellison said that the intense pain of labor made her even more fearful of subsequent pain. In Chapter 3 we mentioned that numerous past experiences with pain tend to cause the individual to perceive pain as threatening and to be more sensitive to such painful stimuli (Collins). This seemed to occur with Mrs. Ellison immediately after one long experience with severe pain. Possibly assistance with assimilating pain would have prevented her "panicked" response to more pain. Thus, when the nurse assists the patient to assimilate pain, she may be preventing a painful experience from having a negative impact upon the patient's ability to deal with future pain.

Mrs. Ellison remained upset about her pain for at least six weeks. This seems to be an unusually long time for an adult to continue to be anxious about an episode of pain, especially when there are no residual complications. However, it is conceivable that more adults remain anxious about a past painful event for a longer time than we realize. We know that children between the ages of two and four years may remain disturbed for up to six months following surgery (Vaughn). Children may be more disturbed by pain and some other aspects of illness than adults, and children may need more assistance with assimilating pain. However, it appears that the adult, too, may be quite upset about pain that has ceased and may require considerable assistance in assimilating an occurrence of pain. Therefore, the assimilation of pain may also serve the purpose of decreasing the incidence, severity or duration of emotional disturbances following pain.

Further Exploration

All the nursing activities for pain relief mentioned in this chapter require further investigation. For that reason this discussion will focus mainly on the contributions that clinical specialists in nursing and nurse-researchers may make in these areas. For many years, nursing identified its specialty areas in the same way as medicine (i.e., pediatric nursing, public health nursing, psychiatric nursing and so on) or in geographic locations in or out of the hospital. More recently, nurses have identified speciality areas more or less in terms of behavioral concepts or disruptions in patient behavior. The nurse may specialize, for example, in the care of the patient with a body image disturbance or the care of the dying patient and his family. Others have identified speciality areas on the basis of intervention strategies. Thus, there are now nurses who specialize in crisis intervention or behavior modification.

There is growing interest in the care of patients with a particular type of problem regardless of where the patients are placed in or out of the hospital and sometimes irrespective of their ages. Such an approach was adopted for this book—the focus is on the care of patients with all types of pain, in any setting and of any age. It seems only logical that the care of the patient with pain is worthy of being considered as a speciality area for the practitioner or the researcher. To go a step further, the nurse might specialize in certain aspects of the management of the patient with pain. She could focus on a certain age group such as children, a particular type of pain such as chronic pain, or one of the nursing activities for pain relief such as providing sensory input of various types. Many of the references in this book indicate that researchers and practitioners in nursing are already concentrating their energies on some specific aspect of the care of the patient with pain.

Both the clinicial specialist and the nurse-researcher may contribute to the body of knowledge about the care of the patient with pain. Broadly speaking, there are three equally important approaches to the study of this subject.

Analysis of techniques of pain relief. One is to determine the relationship between certain characteristics of the patient and the effectiveness of a particular pain relief measure. Undoubtedly some types of patients respond better to certain pain relief measures than to others. And, for some patients, a particular pain relief measure may not only be ineffective but may in fact be harmful.

Many studies have indicated that the patient's personality is a determining factor in his response to a pain relief measure. However, selected psychological tests are frequently used to measure the personality characteristics. In clinical practice it is rare to find a patient who has been tested in this way, and the practitioner usually lacks either the time or the skill to administer such tests. For studies of this kind to have practical value in the actual nursing care of the patient, the results of psychological testing must be correlated with behaviors that can be easily and reliably observed by the practicing nurse. Or, the problem may be studied by relying only on easily observable behaviors or patient characteristics such as age and sex and attempting to correlate them with the effectiveness of a selected pain relief measure.

A second approach to the study of patients with pain is to determine the relationship between certain types of pain and the effectiveness of a particular pain relief measure. For example, it seems rather likely that certain pain relief measures may be more effective with chronic pain than pain of brief duration. Others may be more effective with a moderate intensity of pain than with a very high intensity of pain. That is, the effectiveness of any pain relief measure may be determined in part by the characteristics of the pain.

A third approach to the investigation of pain relief is to determine whether or not a particular variation of a pain relief measure produces greater pain relief or is effective with more people than some other variation of the pain relief measure. For example, with WIA is it more effective to have the patient imagine insensitivity of a painful part or to have him imagine a pleasant sensation? Or, is imagining insensitivity of the painful part effective with fewer patients than imagining a pleasant sensation? In other words, it is possible that imagining insensitivity is more effective than imagining a pleasant sensation, but imagining insensitivity may not be possible for as many people as is imagining a pleasant sensation.

Two nursing activities for pain relief were omitted in this chapter. These are hypnotic anesthesia or analgesia and the use of films or video tapes for teaching patients about pain. Hypnosis was not included because its proper usage involves considerable discussion and experience. It probably should be explored initially by nurses prepared at the masters or doctoral level. Although hypnosis should be employed only under the supervision of a physician, there appears to be no reason why nurses cannot be one of several professional groups educated and skilled in the use of hypnosis as a technique for achieving pain relief. The technique of hypnotic induction may be learned in a very short period of time. It is what the hypnotist says and does during the hypnotic trance that requires great understanding and skill. But, the nurse at the masters or doctoral level could conceivably achieve this degree of understanding and skill.

The study of hypnosis is valuable to nursing not only because the technique can be used to produce pain relief through relaxation, anesthesia or analgesia, but also because the study of hypnosis is one way of examining various principles underlying other pain relief measures. Understanding of and experience with the application of these principles can be gained through the use of hypnosis. This knowledge probably will contribute more to the care of patients with pain than will the actual use of hypnosis. The study of hypnotic analgesia is particularly relevent to the use of WIA. WIA is quite similar to hypnotic analgesia, but it can be used on a broader scale by the beginning practitioner because it does not require skill in hypnotic induction. Further, precipitation of an emotional disturbance is a potential danger during hypnotic trance, but it is not likely to occur with WIA. Thus, the study of hypnosis may lead to the more effective use of WIA. This is important because WIA is a pain relief measure that can be used by people who have no skill with or understanding of hypnosis, and it can be applied without the risks associated with hypnosis. But the value of studying hypnotic analgesia is not limited to the contributions this may make to the use of WIA.

Hypnotic analgesia or anesthesia, and perhaps WIA, can be produced in only a small percentage of the population. However, the principles underlying hynosis may be effectively utilized with a large number of patients in other ways. In this respect, Sternbach's (1968) conclusion after his review of the literature on hypnotic analgesia is of particular interest to nursing. He suggests that in hypnotic analgesia the single necessary and sufficient condition for perceiving a stimulus as a nonpainful sensation is the absence of anxiety about the stimulation. Many pain relief measures besides hypnotic analgesia rely upon the principle of anxiety reduction. Therefore, the study of hypnosis may contribute significantly to the effectiveness of many other pain relief measures.

The use of films, video tapes and other programmed audiovisual instruction for teaching patients about pain was omitted earlier in this chapter because, to this author's knowledge, no such material has been prepared. This method would not replace the need for individual teaching or patient group discussions about pain, but in some ways it probably would be a more efficient and effective teaching method than individual or group instruction. For example, a videotape could be prepared about a particular hospital. It could include a general introduction to the hospital setting and personnel and an explanation of various routines. This might decrease the need to conduct tours of the hospital and explain routines to each patient. A film could be made that demonstrates various equipment associated with painful experiences and certain pain relief measures such as proper positioning and relaxation. Such tapes or films would conserve the nurse's time and energy. In terms of patient care it would mean that all patients would be able to see certain equipment and areas of the hospital that might not always be available for viewing. Also, some pain relief measures such as positioning are better understood by the patient if he can see them performed.

Chapter 6

Evaluation of the Effectiveness of Nursing Intervention

Evaluation of nursing intervention is a two-part process. It involves the nurse's performance on the one hand and the patient's behavioral reactions on the other. Evaluation of the nurse's performance is usually for the purpose of determining whether or not intervention was based upon knowledge and understanding of the patient and certain scientific theories and principles. Part of the evaluation of the nurse is concerned with the nurse-centered objectives mentioned at the beginning of Chapter 5. These are statements in which the nurse describes objectively what she should do for a particular patient. When the nurse formulates and carries out appropriate nurse-centered objectives, she is applying her knowledge and understanding of the patient and the principles of nursing intervention. This suggests that the nurse's intervention was theoretically sound, but it does not necessarily mean that the intervention was effective for the individual patient. It is another matter to evaluate the effectiveness of the care the nurse gives the patient.

Evaluation of the patient's behavioral responses to intervention is for the purpose of determining its effectiveness. This is related in part to the patient-centered objectives mentioned in Chapter 5. These objectives are statements that set forth the nurse's expectations of the patient's behavior in response to her intervention. If the patient responds in the expected way, the nurse knows that the intervention is effective.

Evaluation of both the nurse's behavior and the patient's behavior is important to the process of nursing care. Both enable the nurse to improve her ability to design and implement effective nursing care. It is not enough to say that the nurse understands certain principles of nursing intervention and applies them to the care of the patient. We must go a step further. We must ask, was the intervention effective?

This chapter will focus on various aspects of evaluating the effectiveness of nursing intervention and on how the results of this evaluation help the nurse to maintain or improve the effectiveness of her intervention for the particular patient.

How does the nurse determine objectively the effectiveness of her intervention?

The only way to determine objectively the effectiveness of nursing intervention designed to provide pain relief is to assess the patient's behavioral responses to it. It was previously mentioned that problem-solving is a circular process. This is clearly demonstrated in the problem-solving step of evaluation. Once the nurse has intervened she must begin again to assess the patient's behaviors in essentially the same manner as she did initially. However, this time she compares this new assessment with her initial assessment. If both include objective descriptions of the patient's behavior, a comparison will result in an objective measure of the effectiveness of the nursing intervention.

Table 2 (pp. 206-207) shows how a nurse may organize her assessments of the patient. This method of organization facilitates comparing the initial assessment of the patient with the assessment following intervention. The patient used to illustrate this approach to evaluation is Mr. Brook, 46 years old. He was admitted because of increased pain associated with a malignant and inoperable brain tumor. The physician was attempting to determine the extent of metastasis of the tumor and was considering radiation therapy. The malignancy had been diagnosed six months earlier, and Mr. Brook was told at that time that his illness was terminal. The nurse assigned to Mr. Brook on the second day of his hospitalization assessed his behavioral responses to pain. She assessed each of the categories of behavioral response listed in Column 1 of Table 2. (These categories are discussed in Chapter 2.) The result of this initial assessment of Mr. Brook is recorded in Column 2. The assessment encompasses responses to the second phase of pain, the presence of pain. Mr. Brook experienced almost constant pain. However, the phases of anticipation and aftermath did exist for Mr. Brook in terms of severe pain. At times he anticipated that his pain would increase in intensity from moderate to severe. After the analgesic, he experienced relief from the severe pain. This could be considered the aftermath of severe pain. The nurse did assess Mr. Brook's behavioral responses to the anticipation and aftermath phases of severe pain; however, to make this example as brief and clear as possible, this aspect of her assessment is not included in Column 2.

After her initial assessment of Mr. Brook's behavioral responses to pain the nurse began to determine possible pain relief measures. Mr. Brook explained that he did not want to take analgesics because they affected his ability to think clearly. He said that he knew his tumor might eventually affect his thought processes, and therefore, wanted to think clearly for as long as possible. He especially did not want to take analgesics during the day. The nurse used this information and her assessment of the factors that influenced Mr. Brook's perception and response to pain to determine an overall goal for her intervention: to decrease the perceived intensity of pain and increase pain tolerance. Two of her patient-centered objectives were (1) to decrease the number of times between 7 a.m. and 9 p.m. that Mr. Brook rated his pain as severe and (2) to eliminate Mr. Brook's request for an analgesic between 7 a.m. and 9 p.m. The nurse discussed with Mr. Brook these objectives and her overall goal. He agreed that these were the aspects of pain relief he desired most and that they were the most realistic for him. The nurse later used the overall goal and the patient-centered objectives to determine whether or not her intervention was effective.

The nurse next discussed several pain relief measures with Mr. Brook and taught him how to use those that he wanted to try. Those that he learned and tried the first day were relaxation, distraction and cutaneous stimulation. He used each of these separately and at a time when he rated his pain as moderate in intensity.

After the nurse begins a new program of intervention, there are essentially two ways in which she assesses behavioral responses to it. First she assesses the patient's responses to each aspect of intervention. This assessment is done at several intervals following or during the use of each pain relief measure. Column 3 of Table 2 shows one of the nurse's assessments for each of three aspects of her nursing intervention. Mr. Brook's responses to each of these pain relief measures were assessed separately after the first time he used them. His responses to relaxation and distraction were assessed at several intervals while he was using them. Only the assessment done about one half hour after he began to use each of these is recorded in Column 3. His responses to cutaneous stimulation were also assessed at several intervals after the nurse rubbed his forehead and upper back for three minutes. In Column 3 only the assessment done one half hour after cutaneous stimulation is recorded. In the case of Mr. Brook there are other aspects of nursing intervention that are also pertinent to evaluate in Column 3. These include teaching the patient about pain and establishing a relationship with him. The nurse did these things, but an evaluation of them is omitted here for the sake of brevity.

The second way in which the nurse assesses the behavioral responses to nursing intervention is to assess the total effect of all aspects of intervention for the entire period of time in which the pain experience occurs. For Mr. Brook this total period of time was 24 hours a day. Therefore, on each of the three days following the new program of

TABLE 2.

EVALUATION OF THE EFFECTIVENES[

COLUMN 1 CATEGORIES OF BEHAVIORAL RESPONSE	COLUMN 2 MR. BROOK'S BEHAVIORAL RESPONSES TO PAIN PRIOR TO THE NURSING INTERVENTION IN COLUMN 3	RELAXATION
1. Physiological manifestations	For 6 to 8 hours a day when he experiences moderate pain his vital signs are: P = 80 to 90 R = 14 to 18 BP = 138/108 to 144/116 For about 4 hours a day when he experiences severe pain his vital signs are: P = 90 to 100 R = 16 to 20 BP = 142/114 to 150/120 He is never free of pain. However, vital signs associated with moderate and severe pain may be compared with those following an analgesic, the only time pain does not "bother" him: P = 70 to 80 R = 12 to 14 BP = 136/100 to 140/110 With severe pain his face is slightly pale with perspiration on the forehead.	P = 80 R = 12 BP = 138/96 No pallor or perspiration
2. Verbal statements	When he requests an analgesic he rates his pain as severe. This occurs three times a day, once between 7 a.m. and 9 p.m. and twice between 9 p.m. and 7 a.m. When he has pain but does not want an analgesic, he rates his pain as moderate. He mentions this pain only upon questioning. He seems to experience moderate pain 6 to 8 hours a day. Following an analgesic he states his pain does not "bother" him and that he is drowsy. He usually sleeps about 4 hours after each analgesic. States his pain is "in the back of my neck and goes all the way up to the top of my head." He says it "aches mostly with some sharp, shooting pain." Sometimes the pain increases in intensity when he turns his head from side to side.	When asked he rates his pain as moderat intensity
3. Vocalizations	With severe pain he moans very quietly every 10 to 15 seconds. With moderate pain he makes a quiet grunting noise every few minutes.	No moaning A quiet grunting sound about every 7 minutes.
4. Facial expressions	With severe pain he wrinkles his forehead and clenches his jaws. With moderate pain he clenches his jaws for a few seconds every 5 to 10 minutes.	Facial muscles are relaxed.
5. Amount and type of body movement	With severe pain he makes a tight fist and maintains this constantly. With moderate pain he clenches his fist every few seconds. With both moderate and severe pain his extremities are constantly tense. He is relaxed after an analgesic.	Entire body is relaxed.
6. Physical contact with others	Does not initiate physical contact with others except his wife. With his wife physical contact appears to be an expression of affection not a response to pain. Passively accepts being touched by the nurse.	No change.
7. General response to the environment	Initiates conversation with the nurse and his wife, his only visitor. His roommate is comatose. When he is alone he lies in bed and stares blankly at the T.V. Questioning reveals that he usually does not know what is happening on the T.V. program.	No change. Eyes closed.
8. Pattern of handling pain.	Minimally expressive responses to pain. Attempts to tolerate pain until it becomes severe. Attempts to try to depend upon himself in handling pain. Asks for an analgesic only when he is unable to handle the pain himself. Does not ask for other pain relief measures.	No change.

TABLE 2.

COLUMN 3		COLUMN 4
MR. BROOK'S BEHAVIORAL RESPONSES ONE HALF HOUR AFTER EACH OF THE FOLLOWING ASPECTS OF NURSING INTERVENTION WAS IMPLEMENTED: (EACH WAS USED SEPARATELY AND WHEN PAIN WAS MODERATE)		MR. BROOK'S BEHAVIORAL RESPONSES TO PAIN AFTER THREE DAYS OF USING THE NURSING INTERVENTION IN COLUMN 3
DISTRACTION	CUTANEOUS STIMULATION	
= 88 = 16 = 140/110	P = 70 R = 14 BP = 136/90	For 3 hours a day between 7 a.m. and 9 p.m. when he experiences mild pain without the aid of an analgesic his vital signs are: P = 70 to 80 R = 12 to 16 BP = 132/90 to 140/108 Vital signs for moderate pain, severe pain, and the period following the analgesic are essentially within the same range as they were in the initial assessment. Vital signs typical of severe pain occur 2 hours a day, between 9 p.m. and 7 a.m.; those typical of moderate pain, 8 to 10 hours a day between 7 a.m. and 9 p.m.
pallor or spiration	No pallor or perspiration	Perspiration on the forehead and slight pallor occur about twice for 30 minutes between 9 p.m. and 7 a.m.
n asked he rates his pain as moderate in nsity. However, he says that distraction s his mind "off the pain" so pain no longer hers" him.	Voluntarily comments that his pain is less than moderate but more than mild	For 3 days he has requested an analgesic only twice during each 24 hours. These requests occurred only between 9 p.m. and 7 a.m. At the time he requests an analgesic he rates his pain as severe. He rates his pain as mild for a total of 3 hours each day; moderate, 8 to 10 hours; severe, 2 hours. He has severe pain only between 9 p.m. and 7 a.m. His response following an analgesic remains the same. His description of the location and quality of his pain remains the same.
vocalizations	No vocalizations	Between 7 a.m. and 9 p.m. no moaning occurs. A quiet grunting sound may occur every 10 to 15 minutes. Both moaning and grunting occur between 9 p.m. and 7 a.m. prior to an analgesic.
aches his jaws for a few seconds every 10 utes	Facial muscles are relaxed	Between 7 a.m. and 9 p.m. he may wrinkle his forehead once or twice. Clenching of the jaws may occur every 30 minutes to an hour Between 9 p.m. and 7 a.m. wrinkling of the forehead and clenching of the jaws occurs prior to an analgesic.
nches his fist every few minutes. Otherwise xed except for purposeful movements.	Entire body relaxed. Occasionally rubs his forehead as the nurse had done.	Between 7 a.m. and 9 p.m. extremities may become tense for a few minutes every 30 minutes to an hour. He rarely clenches his fist; this may occur twice a day. Between 9 p.m. and 7 a.m. he clenches his fist every few minutes prior to an analgesic. Every 10 to 15 minutes while he is awake he rubs his forehead.
change.	No change.	No change.
change.	No change.	No change. When he appears to be engaged in an activity such as watching T.V. or number painting, he can tell someone else what is going on in relation to his activity.
ending to the distraction.	Watching T.V. Told the nurse what he was watching.	
change.	No change.	Continues minimally expressive responses to pain. Utilizes several methods other than analgesics for handling pain. Uses these other methods as a means of handling pain himself. However, every 1 to 2 hours during the day he requests cutaneous stimulation from the nurse.

nursing intervention, the nurse assessed Mr. Brook's behavioral responses for the 24-hour period. This assessment is recorded in Column 4 of Table 2.

Once the nurse has assessed the patient's behavioral responses to nursing intervention she is able to evalute its effectiveness. This evaluation is done by comparing her assessments of behavioral responses to intervention with her initial assessment of behavioral responses prior to intervention. For example, the nurse compares each of the assessments in Column 3 with her initial assessment in Column 2 (Table 2). She also compares her assessment in Column 4 with her assessment in Column 2. The assessments following nursing intervention (Columns 3 and 4) in themselves reveal nothing about the effectiveness of the nurse's intervention. This can be determined only by comparing these assessments with the patient's behavioral responses prior to the nursing intervention.

The information gained by comparing the patient's before-and-after responses to intervention can be demonstrated with Table 2. Mr. Brook's immediate behavioral responses to each pain relief measure, relaxation, distraction, and cutaneous stimulation (Column 3), can be compared with initial data (Column 2). This comparison reveals that relaxation resulted in Mr. Brook's perceiving his pain as moderate. His vital signs were comparable to those associated with moderate pain. Other behavioral responses to moderate pain that did not change with relaxation were physical contact with others, his general response to the environment and his pattern of handling pain. However, in spite of the fact that he rated his pain as moderate following relaxation, some of his responses to this moderate pain changed. He did not make the grunting vocalizations as frequently. His facial expression was relaxed and he did not clench his jaws. His body was relaxed and he did not clench his fist. This comparison suggests that relaxation did not decrease the perceived intensity of pain since he continued to rate his pain as moderate. But relaxation did seem to increase his tolerance for moderate pain. In the categories of vocalizations, facial expressions and amount and type of body movement, his responses to moderate pain were less intense with relaxation than without relaxation.

When the same type of comparison is done with distraction and cutaneous stimulation, the results are somewhat different. These two pain relief measures seem to be more effective than relaxation. Distraction, for example, produced a response comparable to that following an analgesic. When Mr. Brook was distracted, he said his pain did not bother him. This is also his comment following an analgesic. Cutaneous stimulation resulted in his rating the discomfort as less than moderate. Other behavioral responses to cutaneous stimulation also indicate this decrease in the perceived intensity of pain.

After comparing the responses in Column 3 with those in Column 2 the nurse knows the degree of immediate effectiveness of each aspect of her intervention. All three aspects of her intervention with Mr. Brook were effective to some extent. In general the most effective was cutaneous stimulation, and distraction was more effective than relaxation.

The data in Table 2 can also be used to demonstrate the effectiveness of intervention over the total period of the pain experience. When the assessment in Column 4 is compared with the assessment in Column 2, it is clear that the nurse's intervention is effective for part of the time during Mr. Brook's 24-hour-a-day experience with pain. Mr. Brook's behavioral responses to pain between 9 p.m. and 7 a.m. change very little, but those between 7 a.m. and 9 p.m. change considerably. For example, following intervention he began to experience a few hours of mild pain each day between 7 a.m. and 9 p.m. Prior to intervention he always rated his pain as either moderate or severe.

One final aspect of evaluating the effectiveness of nursing intervention is to determine whether or not the overall goals and patient-centered objectives have been achieved—that is, if the nurse accomplished what she set out to do. In Mr. Brook's case the overall goal was to reduce the perceived intensity of pain and to increase pain tolerance. This was achieved for the period of Mr. Brook's pain experience that occurred between 7 a.m. and 9 p.m. Initially he perceived pain as moderate or severe during those hours, but following intervention he perceived it as mild or moderate. His increased tolerance for pain is indicated by several behavioral responses such as his ability to attend to stimuli other than pain and the decreased frequency of muscle tension. One of the patient-centered objectives for Mr. Brook was to decrease the number of times between 7 a.m. and 9 p.m. that he rated his pain as severe. This was accomplished since he no longer experienced severe pain during that period of time. Another patient-centered objective was to eliminate Mr. Brook's request for an analgesic between 7 a.m. and 9 p.m. This too was accomplished.

It is important for the nurse to use all of these methods of evaluating the effectiveness of her intervention because one evaluation may reveal effective intervention while another may not. For example, with Mr. Brook each pain relief measure immediately resulted in behavioral changes indicating that it was somewhat effective. However, although it did not happen with Mr. Brook, it is possible that over a 24-hour period these methods of pain relief may not have eliminated the need for one of the analgesics. In other words, the effects of each pain relief measure may be favorable but still may not significantly alter the total pain experience. On the other hand, a single pain relief measure may not be notably effective, but may become so with time. For example, with

Mr. Brook relaxation did not alter the perceived intensity of pain. However, over a period of hours relaxation might have prevented the pain from becoming severe, or may have enhanced the effectiveness of other pain relief measures. When several pain relief measures are employed over a period of time, pain relief eventually may be greater than it was when each measure was employed separately. Also, one combination of pain relief measures may be more effective than another.

Examination of goals may reveal that the nursing intervention was effective, but not as much as the nurse had hoped. Or, the patient may not have expressed pain relief in the manner the nurse anticipated. In other words, the goal and patient-centered objectives may not have been met. If this is the case, the nurse may do one of two things. Either she can continue her efforts to meet the goal and objectives or she can revise the goal and objectives. As mentioned at the beginning of Chapter 5, it is difficult to state patient-centered objectives for pain relief. Patients respond differently to pain relief. The nurse may expect the patient to indicate pain relief in a certain way, and she may state this in a patient-centered objective. However, her evaluation of the effectiveness of each pain-relief measure and of the total program of nursing intervention may suggest that the patient indicates pain relief by some other behavioral response. Therefore, the nurse will need to revise her patient-centered objectives.

How does the nurse handle certain problems that may arise when she attempts to evaluate the effectiveness of her intervention?

A number of problems may arise when the nurse is attempting to be objective in her evaluation of the effectiveness of her intervention. The following ones will be discussed here: evaluating the effectiveness of nursing intervention for only one episode of pain; choosing a method of obtaining verbal statements to assess pain relief; evaluating the response of sleep; and determining whether or not the nursing intervention is actually the cause of pain relief.

It is not always possible to compare the patient's behavioral responses prior to intervention with those following it. The patient may experience only one episode of pain, such as a bone marrow aspiration. Or the patient may experience several periods of pain, but the nurse may observe only one of these. There is only one situation that does not present a problem in evaluating the effectiveness of nursing intervention for one episode of pain: the patient is experiencing pain when the nurse intervenes. In this case the nurse is able to compare the patient's reactions before and after intervention. But when the nurse prepares the patient for impending pain, such as a myelogram, she does not know how he would have behaved in the absence of pain relief measures, since there is no means for comparison.

In such situations, the nurse may evaluate the effectiveness of her intervention in two limited ways. First, she may ask the patient for his opinion regarding the effectiveness of the pain relief measures. If he did not use them, the nurse knows that she did not design effective intervention. If he used the pain relief measures and felt they were effective, the nurse may conclude only that her actions possibly were correct. But not necessarily so; there are many reasons why the patient may claim that the pain relief methods were effective when in actuality they were not. For example, he may have experienced less pain than he expected. However, his expectations may have been unrealistic.

A second means of evaluation in single-episode cases is to compare the patient's response with those of other patients with whom the nurse did not intervene. This is quite unreliable since individuals respond to pain and pain relief in different ways. Nevertheless, if the nurse observes the behavioral responses of many patients to a particular type of pain, she may eventually be able to make tentative conclusions about the effectiveness of her intervention for an individual patient.

Another problem encountered in evaluating the effectiveness of nursing intervention is that of choosing a method of obtaining verbal statements to assess pain relief. There are at least three methods to choose from. The first method, mentioned in Chapter 2, consists of asking the patient to rate the intensity of his pain on a scale. This scale may be composed of five parts: no discomfort, slight (or mild) discomfort, moderate discomfort, severe (or intense) discomfort and very severe (or very intense) discomfort. There are several other variations of this scale that are equally useful (Loan and Dundee, 1967 a and b). Whichever scale is chosen should be used consistently with the same patient. For example, the nurse should not use the word "mild" one time and the word "slight" the next time if these two words are to mean the same thing. If the patient is able to use a scale, he should be asked to rate his pain prior to intervention and at intervals following intervention. Comparison of these ratings of the pain will indicate whether pain decreases, increases or remains the same. This is one way of evaluating the effectiveness of nursing intervention using the patient's verbal statements.

A second method of obtaining verbal statements to assess pain relief following nursing intervention is concerned with the degree to which pain bothers the patient. Both before and after nursing intervention the nurse may ask the patient to rate the extent to which his pain bothers him. For example, the nurse may ask the patient if his discomfort bothers him not at all, a little bit, some, quite a bit or a lot. This method may reveal pain relief when the first method, rating the intensity of pain, does not. Sometimes a pain relief measure such as a narcotic analgesic or distraction does not decrease the perceived intensity of pain—it merely renders the pain less bothersome to the patient.

A third type of scale may be used only following nursing intervention. Instead of asking the patient to rate the severity of his pain or the degree to which pain bothers him, the nurse may ask him to rate the degree of pain relief. There are several different scales of this general type. The nurse may ask the patient to rate his pain relief in any of the following ways: complete, moderate, slight, none; 100%, more than 50%, less than 50%, none; excellent, good, fair, poor, none (Loan and Dundee, 1967 a and b). Again, the nurse should use the same scale consistently with the patient. This type of scale will reveal whether or not any pain relief was achieved through nursing intervention, and also the degree. This type of scale may be somewhat more loosely interpreted by the patient than the other two methods mentioned above. The patient may interpret pain relief as referring either to the intensity of pain or to the degree to which the pain bothers him. He will usually choose the interpretation that is most important and acceptable to him. The disadvantage of rating the degree of pain relief is that it requires a retrospective analysis by the patient. He must be able to compare how he felt before and after nursing intervention. For this reason, rating pain relief is probably less reliable than having the patient rate before and after intervention the intensity of pain or the degree to which pain bothers him. With these latter methods the nurse makes the comparison rather than the patient.

It is usually advisable for the nurse to choose only one of these three methods of obtaining verbal statements to assess pain relief. Most patients with pain find the use of all three methods rather tiresome. If all three were used, the patient would have to rate his pain on two scales prior to intervention and on three scales at intervals following it.

Since there are advantages and disadvantages to each of the methods it is difficult to advise the nurse as to which is the best one. Some patients describe their pain in terms of intensity while others talk more about how bothersome the pain is. A preponderance of either of these comments by a patient suggests the method the nurse should choose for him. Otherwise, to a certain extent the nurse initially may simply use the one she personally prefers.

If the patient has difficulty with the rating scale chosen by the nurse, she may ask him if other items or methods would be easier and more descriptive. It is also possible that a patient will experience different types of pain relief following different pain relief measures. For example, Mr. Brook, described in Table 2, experienced a decreased intensity of pain with cutaneous stimulation. When he used distraction he did not experience a decreased intensity, but he found the pain less bothersome. When this type of situation occurs with a patient the nurse may use different methods for different pain relief measures. Another approach to this situation is to use the method of assessing the degree of pain relief. If the patient says he experiences some degree of pain relief following intervention, the nurse may then ask if the pain is less intense or less bothersome. The patient simply chooses between these two types of pain relief. Unless the patient is interested in doing so, the nurse should not tire him by asking him to rate his answer on another scale.

Regardless of the method the nurse uses to obtain verbal statements to assess pain relief, she should realize that the degree of effectiveness of a pain relief measure is often related to the severity of pain prior to the intervention. Patients who rate their pain as severe or very severe prior to intervention tend to obtain only partial relief following intervention. For example, following intervention they may say that the pain intensity has decreased to moderate or that the pain relief is less than 50 percent. Complete pain relief tends to occur more often with patients who rate their pain as mild or moderate prior to intervention (Lasagna, Laties and Dohan). Therefore, the nurse should not be too disappointed if the patient with very severe pain does not report complete pain relief. Occasionally the patient with severe or very severe pain reports complete pain relief immediately following intervention. However, a few minutes to an hour later he may state that some pain is still present. It has been suggested that this may be due to the immediate emotional relief that accompanies relief from severe pain. Following intervention the pain may be considerably less intense or more tolerable. At first it may seem to the patient that the pain is completely gone. Some time may elapse before the patient perceives that a degree of pain is present (Wolff and Horland).

Still another problem may arise when the nurse evaluates the effectiveness of her intervention. This is the question of what it means when the patient sleeps following a pain relief measure. It is common practice to consider this as a sign of pain relief. Pain may be fatiguing, and it is understandable that the patient might sleep when he is relieved of the pain. However, sleep does not necessarily indicate pain relief. Even the patient with severe pain may sleep. When he is awakened he complains of severe pain. Or, the patient may appear to be asleep because he is motionless with his eyes closed. When certain analgesics are administered the occurrence of sleep has another possible meaning: a side effect of the analgesic. The analgesic may produce drowsiness and sleep without relieving pain.

There are two ways to handle the problem of interpreting the occurrence of sleep following a pain relief measure. First, the nurse may consider sleep a form of pain relief because the patient is not conscious of pain during sleep. Based on this interpretation the nurse may evaluate a pain relief measure as somewhat effective if it produces sleep in a patient who hitherto was unable to do so. However, there is a second and better way of dealing with the occurrence of sleep following a pain relief measure. The nurse simply should make every effort to assess pain relief before the patient goes to sleep.

One particular problem always arises when the nurse attempts to evaluate objectively the effectiveness of her intervention: determining whether or not the nursing intervention is actually the cause of pain relief. That pain relief follows nursing intervention does not necessarily mean that it resulted from the measure. It is not easy to rule out other possible causes of pain relief, but the nurse must be alert to their existence.

In the section on administering placebos in Chapter 5, mention was made of some reasons a patient may report or experience pain relief following a placebo. Essentially these same reasons apply to pain relief following any nursing intervention. Three of these will be discussed again here in a slightly broader context. First, pain relief measures that the nurse is not aware of, not of her instigation, may have been employed at about the same time as her nursing intervention. For example, the nurse tried cutaneous stimulation with Miss Bruce. The nurse then left the room for 15 minutes. During that time Miss Bruce received a telephone call that distracted her from the pain. After the telephone conversation had ended the nurse returned, not knowing about the telephone call. When Miss Bruce reported pain relief, the nurse believed the pain relief resulted only from the cutaneous stimulation. In this situation it is obvious that distraction could have had more to do with pain relief than the cutaneous stimulation. Had the nurse asked Miss Bruce what had happened during her absence, she may have noted this possibility. However, the patient is not always aware of other causes of pain relief and may not report them upon questioning. Therefore, the nurse simply must employ and assess the effectiveness of a particular pain relief measure more than once.

Secondly, pain relief following a particular measure may be due to spontaneous fluctuations in pain intensity. Such fluctuations occur in the normal course of many diseases. Or, pain relief may be due to the process of wound healing. Again, to rule out these possibilities, the nurse must use and evaluate a pain relief measure more than once.

Thirdly, following nursing intervention the patient may deliberately and consciously fake pain relief. To reward the nurse for her attempts to help him, the patient may assure her that her efforts were successful. To detect this the nurse must not only use and evaluate the pain relief measure again, but also look for other signs of pain relief. For example, she may observe that the patient's extremities continue to be tense although he reports pain relief.

How does the nurse utilize her evaluation of the effectiveness of her intervention?

The nurse's evaluation of the effectiveness of her intervention measures may reveal that she has helped the patient achieve as much pain relief as it seems realistic to expect. She should continue their use, but also subject them to constant testing. In addition, she continues to assess factors that influence the patient's behavioral responses to pain and the pain sensation. The patient's pain experience is not static; it may change from day to day or week to week. The factors influencing his behavioral responses and the pain sensation may vary considerably. Hence a pain relief measure may cease to be effective after a period of time. Therefore, it is important for the nurse to continue certain aspects of the problem-solving process even after she has devised intervention that is effective for the patient's pain experience.

It is not unusual for the nurse's evaluation of the effectiveness of her intervention to indicate that the desired level of pain relief has not been achieved. The nurse must then modify her approach. For example, the nurse caring for Mr. Brook (Table 2) noted that relaxation used alone was not as effective as distraction or cutaneous stimulation used alone. Since relaxation was somewhat effective, she did not want to suggest that Mr. Brook abandon it. Instead, she suggested that Mr. Brook use relaxation in conjunction with cutaneous stimulation. The nurse then reassessed the effectiveness of this combination (not shown in Table 2), and found that the combination was more effective than either of its elements used separately.

The nurse's evaluation of the effectiveness of her intervention may or may not indicate the types of modifications she should make. In either case, however, she begins again to go through the steps of problem solving. First, she obtains a new assessment of the patient's behavioral responses to the pain experience. Second, she reassesses the factors that influence the patient's behavioral responses and the pain sensation. She states another nursing diagnosis. She proceeds again to devise nursing intervention. And once more she evaluates the effectiveness of that intervention.

What does it mean when the nurse is unable to design effective nursing intervention for a patient with pain?

Before the nurse decides she is unable to design effective nursing intervention for a patient, she should do two things. First, she should go through the process of problem solving more than once. Many times it is necessary to modify, delete or add to her initial efforts at providing pain relief. Secondly, she should re-examine her goals and objectives.

The nurse's intervention may appear to be ineffective if she has stated unrealistic goals and patient-centered objectives. For example, if one of the patient-centered objectives for Mr. Brook (Table 2) had been to eliminate the need for all analgesics, the intervention would appear to be ineffective. The nurse must carefully set realistic goals that are acceptable and desirable to the patient. Otherwise both will feel an unjustified sense of failure.

But, what is wrong when the goals of pain relief are realistic and the nurse fails to devise effective nursing intervention after repeated attempts? There are innumerable possibilities. A few of the more common reasons for failure will be discussed here. However, the nurse should not use any of these reasons as an excuse for ceasing to exert her fullest efforts to assist the patient with pain.

Sometimes the nurse's repeated attempts at providing pain relief are ineffective because she is overlooking something. Perhaps she has not systematically tried to determine the presence or absence of all the factors that may influence the patient's responses to pain or the pain sensation. She must investigate more closely. For example, after several attempts the nurse was still unable to provide an effective degree of pain relief for Mrs. Harper who had a gastric ulcer. She then made a list of the influencing factors discussed in Chapter 3. She began observing more closely and asking Mrs. Harper more questions. At one point she decided to find out more about whether the influence of others who came in contact with Mrs. Harper could be contributing to Mrs. Harper's pain experience. The nurse asked Mrs. Harper whom she saw each day and what they discussed. It happened that Mrs. Harper's son, a medical student, visited every three days. The nurse was aware of these visits, and Mrs. Harper had always said she enjoyed seeing her son. However, the nurse had not realized that the son telephoned every day, and that all the conversations concerned the possibly dire implications of Mrs. Harper's symptoms and disease. Mrs. Harper's son apparently felt he was being helpful by explaining to his mother all of the things that might happen during her illness. Mrs. Harper tried to ignore what her son suggested might occur, and tried to rely upon the statements of her physician. Mrs. Harper said she knew that most of what her son talked about was unlikely to occur in her case, and so had never mentioned the conversations, but nevertheless found it difficult not to think of all the things her discomfort might mean. When the son visited the next day, the nurse discussed with him the effect of this upon his mother. The son immediately resolved to avoid that type of conversation, and Mrs. Harper experienced greater pain relief.

Another reason nursing intervention may be ineffective is that the nurse may not believe in the effectiveness of a pain relief measure, or at least may not be enthusiastic about its usage. It is quite possible that the nurse's best efforts will not succeed in hiding her lack of confidence in the pain relief measure, and the patient may sense this. The negative effect on the patient may be comparable to what occurs in the placebo phenomenon. In the discussion of the placebo in Chapter 5, mention was made of a study in which some patients did not receive pain relief from intravenous morphine when they were told it would be ineffective (Keats). This suggests that if the patient perceives that the nurse does not have confidence in a pain relief measure, he may not benefit from it. There are numerous accounts of the relationship between the physician's enthusiasm and the results of his treatment. For example, when the physician is enthusiastic about a drug, his patients tend to respond more favorably to the drug than the patients of a physician who does not believe in the drug (Wolf). In all likelihood this positive correlation between favorable results and enthusiasm holds true for nursing intervention.

It may be difficult for the nurse to overcome her disbelief in the effectiveness of certain pain relief measures. She may have seen the pain relief measure fail with several patients, or, she may have tried it on herself without success. However, the nurse should try to appreciate the fact that every patient is different. Something that does not provide pain relief for one person may be effective with another.

One other reason the nurse may not be able to provide the desired degree of pain relief is that the patient may be unable to relinquish his pain. In the literature there are many references to the "pain-prone" person. We have already discussed that some people use pain to deal with emotional conflicts; that is, they would rather experience the pain than the emotional problem. Not all of these patients will agree to or benefit from psychiatric help. Hence the pain will persist.

Some of these so-called pain-prone patients seem to invite pain in the form of surgical procedures. They may go from one physician to another and almost demand that a surgical procedure be performed to treat the pain. These patients eventually may undergo an incredible number of operations. Yet pain continues.

There is another type of person who simply has difficulty responding to pain relief measures. He is not necessarily pain-prone, but he habitually responds negatively to pain relief measures. This type of person has been described as having an approach-avoidance conflict in relation to pain relief. To this person pain relief seems to be associated with dependency, passivity and regression. This regression threatens the patient. As a result, the more he desires pain relief the more anxious he becomes. This represents a conflict in which the patient is tempted to obtain pain relief but cannot permit it because of the unacceptable regression. This conflict is most likely to occur in patients who value minimal expression of pain. The patient who experiences the approach-avoidance conflict is often angry, critical and frightened. He is also unlikely to respond to pain relief measures (Sternbach, 1968).

Patients who have difficulty relinquishing their pain, for whatever reason, will not respond well to pain relief measures. The nurse's intervention for them will be ineffective at least part of the time. However, if the nurse continues her efforts she probably will be able to provide some pain relief from time to time.

Finally, the nurse should remember that there is still much to learn about pain relief. What is known to this point may be insufficient for relieving a particular patient's pain. She must be persistent and creative in her efforts, always searching for new answers.

Further Exploration

The type of evaluation of the effectiveness of nursing intervention suggested in this chapter was described in relation to the nurse's care of the individual patient. It was assumed that each nurse caring for each patient with pain should carry out this process of evaluation. However, evaluation can be a time-consuming and tedious task for the busy practicing nurse, essential as it may be. The process can be facilitated by including a form for evaluation in the chart of each patient who experiences pain. This form could be similar to the one used in Table 2.

The type of evaluation described in this chapter may also be of interest to the nurse educator. The form presented in Table 2 can be used as a guide for the student's care and the presentation of her patient care. This method of organizing assessment, intervention and evaluation assists the student to think logically and to gain an appreciation of the usefulness of the process of problem solving.

Some aspects of this type of evaluation may also be useful to the nurse researcher. In nursing research the patient's verbal or written comments are often used to evaluate the effectiveness of a pain relief measure. This is a reasonable method to use with adult patients, but it cannot be used with children who have little facility with language. With the exception of the category of verbalizations, the form for assessment presented in Table 2 may be one method the researcher can employ to evaluate the child's responses to pain relief measures.

In this chapter mention was made again of a difference between the intensity of pain and the extent to which pain bothers the patient. Beecher (1956c) makes a similar distinction that differentiates between comfort and pain relief. He appears to equate pain relief with a decrease in the perceived intensity of pain. He associates comfort with the patient's being content and divorced from the painful experience. Thus, his distinction between types of pain relief seems to be the same as this author's. Further, Beecher feels that there are four categories of responses that may follow a pain relief measure: (1) no comfort, no pain relief; (2) no comfort, pain relief; (3) comfort, no pain relief; and (4) comfort, pain relief. In his opinion only the latter two categories of response represent the desired effect, either being acceptable to both physician and patient. What is most interesting is that pain relief with no comfort apparently is not acceptable to the patient. This is worthy of nursing research. If it is true, then it is more important to assess the degree to which pain bothers the patient than to assess the intensity of pain, and priority should be given to pain relief measures that render pain less bothersome or make the patient more comfortable.

Chapter | 7

Guide for the Nursing Care of a Patient with Pain: Assessment, Diagnosis, Intervention and Evaluation — A Summary

The following guide to the nursing care of the patient with pain summarizes the preceding chapters and may be used as a plan for action in the clinical setting. It applies equally well to both children and adults. Naturally in the care of the individual patient certain aspects of the guide will be more applicable than others.

This guide is presented in outline form and is structured on the problem-solving process set forth in this book. Questions are asked about each step of the problem-solving process as it relates to the patient with pain. Brief comments and listings are included as reminders of some of the pertinent points discussed in the text. For the most part this guide includes only what the nurse actually does in behalf of the patient; theories underlying the nurse's actions are omitted. If the nurse wishes to review the discussion of any aspect of this guide, she may refer to the page numbers in parentheses following the question or comment.

I. What are this patient's *behavioral responses* to his pain experience? (Chapter 1, pp. 5 to 9; Chapter 2, pp. 11 to 26)

Pain is whatever the experiencing person says it is and exists whenever he says it does. What the patient "says" about his pain experience is not limited to his verbal and vocal responses; it encompasses all of his behavioral responses to his pain experience. (pp. 8 to 9)

There are three phases of the pain experience—anticipation, presence and aftermath. The nurse assesses the behavioral responses for each phase experienced by the patient. She should be particularly alert to those behavioral responses that reveal the meaning of pain to the patient, the patient's tolerance for pain and the characteristics of the pain such as intensity, location, duration, quality and rhythmicity. All behavioral responses should be described objectively, including their frequency and duration. The following questions may aid the nurse in making a thorough assessment of the patient's behavioral responses.

A. What are this patient's *physiological manifestations* associated with the pain experience? (pp. 13 to 15)

Assessment should include manifestations characteristic of any of the following:

1. Activation.
2. Rebound.
3. Adaptation.
4. Stress Reaction.

B. What *verbal statements* does this patient make about his pain experience? What is his tone of voice? What is his rate of speech? (pp. 15 to 20)

A vast amount of information can be obtained from the patient who is willing and able to communicate verbally. Whenever possible the nurse should encourage the patient to discuss the following items.

1. The severity of his pain, using a rating scale.
2. His tolerance for pain.
3. Characteristics of his pain such as quality (pricking, aching, etc.) location, duration, rhythmicity.
4. The meaning of pain to the patient, and other factors affecting his pain experience.

Certain factors may influence the presence, severity, and characteristics of the pain sensation or the patient's tolerance for pain.

C. What vocalizations does this patient make during his pain experience? (p. 20)

Vocalizations should be assessed in terms of pitch and volume as well as frequency and duration.

D. What are this patient's *facial expressions* during his pain experience? (p. 20)

These should be assessed in terms of facial appearance such as wrinkling of the skin, opened or closed eyes, position of the lips, etc.

E. What are the characteristics of this patient's *bouy movement* during the pain experience? (pp. 20 to 22)

The following forms of body movement should be assessed:

1. Immobility.
2. Purposeless or inaccurate movements.
3. Protective movements, including voluntary and involuntary

movements and those characteristic of either a fight or flight reaction.

4. Rhythmic or rubbing movements.

F. How does this patient *utilize physical contact with others* during his pain experience? (p. 23)

The following forms of physical contact should be assessed.

1. Fight reactions.
2. Initiation of touch.
3. Passive or active acceptance of touch.

G. What is this patient's *general response to the environment* during his pain experience? (pp. 23 to 24)

Pain tends to draw attention to itself. It is important to note the extent to which the patient attends to aspects of his environment other than those associated with his pain experience.

H. Has the patient developed a *pattern of handling his pain experience?* (pp. 24 to 25)

This pattern may encompass any one or combination of the preceding behavioral responses. Behavioral responses may be considered a pattern if they occur repeatedly.

II. What are the *influencing factors* related to this patient's behavioral responses and to his pain sensation? (Chapter 3, pp. 27 to 68)

There are a number of factors that may affect the patient's behavioral responses to his pain experience and/or affect his pain sensation. Some influencing factors tend to have a rather direct effect on some particular aspect of either the pain sensation or the behavioral responses. Others do not necessarily have a tendency to affect a specific aspect of the pain experience. For each factor brief comments are made with regard to which aspects of the pain experience it is likely to affect. However, because of the interplay between the sensation of pain and the responses to it, each influencing factor eventually affects all aspects of the pain experience. (pp. 27 to 28)

A. What are the *physiological and physical factors* influencing this patient's behavior and the pain sensation? (pp. 27 to 44)

The following are examples of physiological and physical factors:

1. Neurophysiological processes underlying the sensation of pain. (pp. 29 to 36)

This factor should be assessed by determining the intactness of the neuroanatomical structures and pathways, the existence of referred pain, and the mechanisms that may underlie the sensation of pain. These mechanisms may be based on the specificity theory, the pattern theory or the gate control theory. This factor may explain why the patient's specific pathology results in a sensation of pain and why the pain is localized in a certain area of his body.

2. Duration and intensity of pain. (pp. 36 to 38)

The duration of pain may range from brief to chronic. Pain may occur once or several times. The intensity of pain may range from none or mild to very severe. This factor may influence any or all of the patient's behavioral responses to his pain experience. Pain of long duration may cause future pain.

3. Alterations in the level of consciousness. (pp. 38 to 39)

The patient's level of consciousness may be altered by conditions such as head injury, drugs, infections of the central nervous system, and decreased oxygenation of the brain. This factor may influence any or all of the patient's behavioral responses to his pain experience. It may also influence the perceived intensity of the pain sensation.

4. Cutaneous versus visceral sites of pain. (pp. 39 to 40)

The patient's response to pain caused by an external or internal source may also resemble the responses associated with cutaneous or visceral pain, respectively. This factor may influence any or all of the patient's behavioral responses to pain. It may also influence the quality of his pain sensation.

5. Environmental conditions. (pp. 40 to 42)

Various aspects of this factor are solar radiation, strong winds or slight drafts, extreme heat or cold, high or low humidity, high altitudes and air pollution. This factor may cause a pain sensation or increase the intensity of existing pain.

6. Sensory restriction. (pp. 42 to 43)

This factor may take the form of sensory deprivation, perceptual deprivation or perceptual monotony. The presence of any of these may increase the perceived intensity of pain, decrease pain tolerance or increase the number of mild discomforts.

7. Physical strain and fatigue. (pp. 43 to 44)

This factor involves temporary mechanical strain on body parts as well as inadequate sleep or rest. Mechanical strain may cause pain or increase the intensity of pain. Fatigue may influence any or all of the patient's behavioral responses to pain. In particular, fatigue may lead to frightening fantasies about the meaning of the pain. Also, it may decrease the patient's tolerance for pain or alter his method of handling pain.

B. What aspects of this patient and his pain determine the *cultural influences* on his behavioral responses and his pain sensation? (pp. 44 to 52)

1. Membership in a particular sociocultural group. (pp. 45 to 50)

Assessment of this factor involves determining the patient's attitudes and values in relation to his pain and to his behavioral responses. This includes assessing such items as whether the patient is more concerned about the pain sensation itself or the future implications of the pain, whether he values palliative or curative pain relief, and whether or not he has confidence in the health team. This factor may influence any or all of the patient's behavioral responses to pain. It may also affect pain tolerance and the existence or perceived intensity of pain.

2. Age and sex. (p. 50)

In general this factor influences the degree of freedom with which the patient responds to pain. Hence, it may affect any or all of the patient's behavioral responses to his pain experience.

3. Religion. (pp. 50 to 51)

Assessment of this factor involves determining the meaning of pain to the patient in terms of his religious beliefs. For example, pain may mean punishment or identification with God. The nurse also assesses whether or not the patient uses prayer or religious ritual in handling pain. This factor may influence any or all of the patient's behavioral responses to his pain experience.

4. Body part involved in pain. (p. 51)

In assessing this factor the nurse determines whether or not the patient views the body part in which pain is localized as an acceptable and socially acknowledged area of the body. This factor may influence in particular the patient's verbal statements about his pain.

5. Roles ascribed to members of the health team. (pp. 51 to 52)

Assessment of this factor involves determining what the patient expects of each member of the health team. This factor may influence whether or not the patient reports pain to the nurse.

C. What are the *psychological factors* influencing this patient's behavioral responses and the pain sensation? (pp. 52 to 65)

1. Emotionally traumatic life experiences. (pp. 52 to 53)

Assessment of this factor involves determining whether or not an emotional problem or personal unhappiness occurred preceding the onset of pain or preceding an increase in the intensity of pain. This factor may initiate, sustain or increase the intensity of a localized sensation of pain.

2. Secondary gains of the patient's complaint of pain. (p. 54)

To assess this factor the nurse must determine whether the patient's complaint of pain results in his accomplishing a goal that he seems unable to achieve in other ways. This factor may influence any or all of the patient's behavioral responses to his pain experience.

3. Personal past experience with pain. (pp. 54 to 55)

Assessment of this factor involves determining the numbers and types of painful experiences the patient has had, the conditions under which these occurred, and the measures that relieved the patient's pain. The more experience a person has had with pain, the more likely he is to perceive pain as threatening and to be more sensitive to painful stimuli. Thus, this factor may affect any or all of the patient's behavioral responses to his pain experience. It may also affect the presence, intensity and quality of his pain sensation.

4. Knowledge, understanding and cognitive level. (pp. 56 to 59)

In assessing this factor it is especially important to ascertain whether or not the patient has an accurate understanding of when pain will occur, the intensity and duration of the pain, and the implications of the pain. It is also important to find out what he understands about pain relief measures. This factor affects the presence and severity of pain and the meaning of pain to the patient, hence it may influence the pain sensation and any or all of the patient's responses to his painful experience.

5. Powerlessness. (pp. 59 to 60)

Assessment of this factor involves determining whether or not the patient feels he has any control over his pain experience. It may influence the amount of information the patient seeks or retains in relation to his pain experience. Consequently it may affect the meaning of pain to the patient. This means that powerlessness may influence the pain sensation and any or all of the patient's behavioral responses to the pain experience.

6. Presence, attitudes and feelings of others. (pp. 60 to 62)

To assess this factor the nurse must become aware of every person who comes in contact with the patient. She must find out which persons assist the patient with his pain and which do not. Persons who may cause the patient to have a more difficult pain experience are those who are annoyed by the patient's manner of responding to pain, who tell the patient to expect pain but do not offer information on pain relief, and who are anxious or angry in the presence of the patient. These reactions may influence the pain sensation and/or the patient's behavioral responses to the pain experience.

7. Threat to life situation. (pp. 62 to 64)

This factor must be assessed by exploring the meaning of pain to the patient. The patient may feel that pain threatens his life, his manner of living, or his body image. Any threat may influence the pain sensation and/or the patient's responses to the pain experience.

8. Perceptual dominance of pain. (p. 64)

This factor is present if the patient has two pain sensations of unequal intensity or if he has intense pain. Mild pain may not be noticed or may be perceived at a lesser intensity in the presence of more severe pain. Or, one intense sensation of pain may raise the threshold of perception for other sensory inputs such as hearing. As a result, if pain gains perceptual dominance it may influence other pain sensations or the patient's responses to the dominant pain.

9. Basic algesic types. (pp. 64 to 65)

The three basic algesic types are reducers, augmenters and moderates. The patient's algesic type influences his estimation of the intensity of pain. Therefore, this factor may influence the pain sensation and the patient's behavioral responses to pain.

D. What are the *relationships between or the combined effects* of several influencing factors? (pp. 65 to 66)

The nurse determines whether or not two or more influencing factors have a common theme or a combined effect.

III. What is the *nursing diagnosis* for this patient with pain? (Chapter 4, pp. 69 to 76)

The nursing diagnosis is a brief summary and organization of the preceding assessment. This diagnosis should be communicated to others to improve the care the patient receives. The nursing diagnosis is composed of the following four parts.

A. What is the nature of this pain sensation? (p. 70)

This includes such items as the intensity, quality, location, duration and intermittency of the pain sensation.

B. What factors influence the existence and characteristics of this pain sensation? (pp. 70 to 72)

This includes factors that cause the painful sensation and that influence the characteristics mentioned in the preceding Part A.

C. What are this patient's behavioral responses to his pain experience? (pp. 72 to 73)

This includes the patient's response to each phase of the pain experience. The most pertinent, most easily observed and/or most frequently occurring responses should be stated.

D. What factors influence this patient's behavioral responses to his pain experience? (pp. 73 to 74)

This includes factors that help to explain why the patient

responds to his pain experience in the particular manner stated in the preceding Part C. For the sake of brevity and practicality this part of the nursing diagnosis may be limited to factors that are major determinants of the patient's behavior and those that are pertinent to nursing management of pain.

IV. What *nursing intervention* may assist this patient during his pain experience? (Chapter 5, pp. 77 to 202)

Individualized nursing intervention is based upon the nurse's assessment of the patient. Nursing intervention is designed to manage those factors that influence the patient's pain sensation and his behavioral responses to pain. The nurse also designs intervention or approaches that are appropriate ways of responding to the patient's behavioral responses to his pain experience. (pp. 77 to 78)

A. What are the *overall goals* of the nursing intervention for this patient with pain? (p. 78)

These goals are general statements about types of pain relief the nurse expects to provide for the patient. Some examples of such goals are: elimination of pain, decrease in the anxiety occurring during the aftermath phase of pain, decrease in the intensity of pain, and increase in pain tolerance.

B. What are the *patient-centered objectives* of the nursing intervention for this patient's pain experience? (pp. 79 to 81)

These statements objectively describe the patient's behavior that will indicate pain relief.

C. What *nursing activities* may be used to assist this patient *during the anticipation and/or presence of pain?* (pp. 81 to 193)

Several of the following nursing activities should be selected and employed to assist the patient with his pain experience. They are based on the nurse's assessment of the patient. The nurse should be sure that her selection of activities for pain relief enables her to manage as many as possible of the factors that influence the patient's pain sensation and his responses to his pain experience. The nurse should also select nursing activities that enable her to react appropriately to the patient's behavioral responses. (pp. 77 to 78, 83 to 84)

1. Establishing a relationship with this patient with pain. (pp. 84 to 93)

The nurse attempts to convey to the patient that she is concerned about him, that she can be trusted to help him and to believe him, that to the extent possible she wants to comply with his expectations of her and of his total medical management, and that she can help him with the emotional and intellectual aspects of his pain experience as well as the physical aspects. The nurse may accomplish this by maintaining the essential characteristics of the one-person situation; by establishing eye contact with the patient; by using projection or doll play with the child; by discussing and giving care that corresponds with this patient's values and expectations of medical management; by exploring the intellectual, emotional and physical aspects of the meaning of pain to this patient; by accepting this patient's behavioral responses to pain; and by promoting the desired relationship between this patient and someone else when the nurse is unable to establish it.

2. Teaching this patient about pain. (pp. 93 to 108)

This nursing activity may include giving this patient information about when the painful event will occur, how long his pain will last, the quality of the pain sensation, proper terminology for the location of the pain, the safety of the painful situation, the equipment and people associated with the pain, when to report pain, and the availability and effectiveness of pain relief measures. In doing these things the nurse avoids the use of the word "pain," avoids persuading the patient to feel pain, uses a variety of the patient's sensory modalities to convey information, includes what the patient believes will relieve pain or convinces him of the effectiveness of certain pain relief measures, involves the patient in making a decision about what will relieve his pain, makes positive statements about the effectiveness of a pain relief measure, and avoids suggesting further action for pain relief at the time a pain relief measure is administered. When possible, teaching the patient about pain should begin prior to the occurrence of pain and as soon as the patient is aware that he will experience. it.

3. Using the patient group situation. (pp. 108 to 113)

Teaching patients in groups should be considered in any setting where several patients each day need to be taught about similar painful experiences. The size of the group usually should be small, preferably five members including the nurse. Group discussion should be encouraged. It may be appropriate for family members to be part of the group.

4. Managing other people who come in contact with this patient. (pp. 113 to 120)

The nurse's interactions with these people may include encouraging them to continue whatever they are doing that promotes pain relief in the patient, suggesting to them ways they may assist the patient, and alleviating their anxieties or anger related to the patient with pain. When anxieties or anger cannot be alleviated, the nurse may then alter the situation by removing that person from the patient's environment or by postponing a painful event.

5. Providing other sensory input. (pp. 120 to 132)

Two methods of increasing sensory input are (1) distraction and (2) touch or other forms of cutaneous stimulation. The nurse may enhance the effectiveness of distraction as a pain relief measure by maximizing the patient's efforts or active participation in relation to the distraction, by involving two or more sensory modalities, and by getting the patient to keep his eyes open. A normal level and variety of meaningful sensory input may be sufficient to produce pain relief if the patient is exposed to a form of sensory restriction. Touch, such as holding the patient's hand, should be provided if the patient accepts or desires it. The large cutaneous afferent fibers may be stimulated by moderate massage, pressure, vibration, bathing or the application of menthol rubbing agents. The area of the body that should be stimulated to provide pain relief may involve the skin over or surrounding the pain sensation or the area on the opposite side of the body corresponding to the painful site.

6. Promoting rest and relaxation. (pp. 132 to 139)

Various aids to sleep include medications such as sedatives, analgesics or alcoholic beverages; attenuation of noise; and minimizing the number of sleep interruptions especially during REM sleep. Relaxation may be enhanced by general comfort measures, muscle relaxant drugs, and certain techniques that teach the patient to relax in response to pain. The latter includes instructing the patient to breathe deeply and relax on expiration and training him to relax the body while one muscle group is contracted.

7. Using behavior therapy. (pp. 139 to 143)

This nursing activity includes rewarding the patient for learning to use new pain relief measures, or for cooperating with painful activities and thereby preventing further pain. It also includes teaching the patient to make responses to pain that are incompatible with pain responses. An example of this is the Lamaze method of training for childbirth. The Lamaze method may be modified and taught to patients who experience other types of discomfort. To decrease the patient's fear and anxiety about a painful experience, the nurse may employ "shaping" and several forms of desensitization, including "fading in."

8. Administering pharmacological agents. (pp. 143 to 157)

The pain-relieving potential of all drugs should be explained to the patient, stressing either the curative or immediate pain-relieving aspects in accordance with the values the patient places on each of these characteristics. When the patient receives a specific analgesic, one that relieves only a certain type of pain, the nurse should explain that the medication probably will not be effective with other types of pain and that it often replaces the need for nonspecific analgesics. With regard to nonspecific analgesics, the nurse works closely with the physician. She must also exercise considerable judgement in administering p.r.n. analgesics. The following will assist the nurse in carrying out these responsibilities. The potency of nonspecific analgesics should be determined by the intensity of pain the patient perceives and not the degree of pathology involved. Generally the most potent analgesics are narcotics administered parenterally. Addiction is not likely to occur when narcotic injections are given for severe pain over a period of days. Within limits the potency of an analgesic can be adjusted by increasing or decreasing the dosage. Oral analgesics are indicated when absorption from the gastrointestinal tract is adequate and when pain is mild to moderate in intensity. A narcotic given orally is not as potent as the same dosage given parenterally. Aspirin is a relatively safe and potent oral analgesic. Beer or wine with meals may also contribute to pain relief. Analgesics should be given early in the pain experience prior to pain becoming severe. Tranquilizers, antidepressants and sedatives may also be used in the treatment of pain.

9. Administering placebos. (pp. 157 to 170)

The nurse's understanding of the placebo phenomenon helps her to detect a true and positive placebo response, to appreciate the meaning of such a response, and to make appropriate suggestions regarding the use of placebos. The pain relief following a true placebo response is genuine. However, the nurse must assess whether or not a true placebo response has actually occurred. The nurse may suggest to the physician that a placebo is one appropriate method of providing pain relief: (1) when the administration of pain-relieving drugs produces undesirable side effects or possibly may lead to addiction, (2) when a procedure cannot be done in the presence of an analgesic, or (3) when medications and procedures seem to be the only form of communication the patient understands. When a physician prescribes a placebo the nurse must find out what the patient is supposed to believe about the placebo and whether or not the physician intends to inform the patient that he has received a placebo.

10. Using waking-imagined analgesia (WIA). (pp. 170 to 176)

The patient may imagine a generally pleasant or exciting event that distracts him from the pain, or he may imagine a pleasant or nonpainful sensation as a substitute for the painful sensation. It may be particularly helpful if the patient imagines that the source of pain is external to his body and that it is a sensation similar to the discomfort but more acceptable. To enhance the effectiveness of WIA the nurse should adhere to certain principles of introducing and explaining WIA to the patient.

11. Decreasing noxious stimuli. (pp. 176 to 179)

The method the nurse uses to decrease noxious stimuli depends upon the patient's particular pathology. Examples of several methods and principles are given in the text.

12. Utilizing other professional assistance. (pp. 179 to 189)

Numerous professional groups may make significant contributions to the management of the patient with pain. The nurse should utilize them to provide the maximum degree of pain relief. It is especially important to seek the assistance of other professional groups whenever the nurse is repeatedly unable to provide a reasonable and satisfactory level of pain relief for the patient. The text discusses the contributions of social workers, clergymen, anesthesiologists and psychiatrists. Comments are also made regarding the use of hypnosis.

13. Being with the patient. (pp. 190 to 193)

During any of the phases of pain the patient may desire the simple presence of the nurse. If the nurse is unable to stay with the patient, she should come to his bedside at frequent and regular intervals, telling the patient when he can expect her to return. In addition she may enlist a volunteer or family member to remain with the patient.

D. What *nursing activities* may be used to assist this patient during the aftermath of pain? (pp. 193 to 200)

Any of the nursing activities suggested in the preceding Part C may be appropriate during the aftermath of pain. The following activities are specific to the aftermath phase of the pain experience.

1. Conveying that the source of noxious stimuli has been removed or decreased. (pp. 194 to 196)

This does not mean that the nurse tells the patient that his pain has ceased. Rather, she tells him when something has been done to diminish or eliminate a cause of his pain. This is particularly relevant following a diagnostic or therapeutic procedure since the patient may not realize the procedure has ended. Adults may be informed verbally; a child may require distraction or cuddling.

2. Assisting with the assimilation of the painful experience. (pp. 196 to 200)

The nurse encourages the patient to express what he remembers about the characteristics of the painful sensations, his emotions and thoughts during his pain, his overt responses to the pain, and what other people were doing and saying during his pain. This may be done verbally with the adult; with the child it may be accomplished through doll play. The nurse should be alert to the patient's need for additional knowledge about his painful experience and his need for praise and reassurance. It may be helpful if the patient, child or adult, keeps a souvenir of the painful event.

V. What is revealed in the *evaluation* of the effectiveness of nursing intervention for this patient? (Chapter 6, pp. 203 to 218)

Evaluation is based upon certain methods of examining the patient's responses to nursing intervention. Evaluation indicates, at least in general, what the nurse should do to maintain or enhance the effectiveness of her intervention for the particular patient.

A. How effective is *each pain relief measure* used with this patient? (pp. 204 to 210)

The patient's behavioral responses to pain relief measures are assessed at intervals following or during the use of each. These behavioral responses are compared with those shown prior to the pain relief measure.

B. How effective is the *total program of nursing intervention* for relieving this patient's pain? (pp. 204 to 210)

The nurse assesses the patient's behavioral responses for the total period of time in which he experiences pain. This should be done for several of these periods of time. These responses are compared with the patient's behavioral responses to a complete episode of pain prior to nursing intervention.

C. Has nursing intervention to assist this patient with his pain experience accomplished the *overall goals and patient-centered objectives*? (pp. 204 to 210)

The results of the preceding Parts A and B are compared with the goals and patient-centered objectives stated prior to nursing intervention.

D. Have certain *problems* arisen that need to be handled in order to regard the evaluation as objective and reliable? (pp. 210 to 214)

The nurse should detect and attempt to handle the following common problems: evaluating the effectiveness of only one episode of pain for which the nurse prepared the patient in advance, choosing a method of obtaining verbal statements to assess pain relief, evaluating the response of sleep following pain relief measures, and determining whether or not the nursing intervention is actually the cause of pain relief.

E. What does the nurse's evaluation *suggest should be done* for this patient? (p. 215)

If the nurse is effective, she continues to employ the effective pain relief measures. Because the patient's pain experience is not static, she also continues to evaluate the effectiveness of her intervention and to assess the factors that may influence the patient's behavioral responses and his pain sensation.

If the nursing intervention does not achieve the desired degree of pain relief, the nurse modifies her intervention. Her evaluation may indicate which pain relief measure should be changed or deleted. In addition, the nurse further modifies her intervention by resuming the entire process of problem solving.

The inability to devise effective intervention may occur because the nurse has overlooked some influencing factors or some pain relief measure. Repeating the process of problem solving in a more systematic way may remedy this problem. Ineffective intervention may also be due to the patient's being unable to relinquish his pain. Finally, nursing intervention may be ineffective because we simply do not yet know enough to help every single patient. In any event, the nurse should continue her efforts to provide as much pain relief as possible. (pp. 215 to 218)

References

1. Abbott, N. C., Hensen, P., and Lewis, K.: Dress rehearsal for the hospital. Am. J. Nurs., 70:2360, 1970.
2. Alexander, L.: Differential diagnosis between psychogenic and physical pain. JAMA, 181:149, 1962.
3. Armstrong, D., et al.: Pain-producing substance in human inflammatory exudates and plasma. J. Physiol., 135:350, 1957.
4. Bandler, R. J., Jr., Madaras, G. R., and Bem, D. J.: Self-observation as a source of pain perception. J. Personality Soc. Psychol., 9:205, 1968.
5. Barber, T. X.: Hypnosis, analgesia, and the placebo effect. JAMA, 172:680, 1960.
6. Barber, T. X., and Hahn, K. W., Jr.: Physiological and subjective responses to pain-producing stimulation under hypnotically-suggested and waking-imagined "analgesia." J. Abnorm. Soc. Psychol., 65:411, 1962.
7. Batterman, R. C.: Clinical aspects of the evaluation of analgesic agents. JAMA, 155:965, 1954.
8. Beecher, H. K.: Limiting factors in experimental pain. J. Chronic. Dis., 4:11, 1956. (a)
9. Beecher, H. K.: Relationship of significance of wound to pain experienced. JAMA, 161:1609, 1956. (b)
10. Beecher, H. K.: The subjective response and reaction to sensation. Am. J. Med., 20:107, 1956. (c)
11. Beecher, H. K.: Generalization from pain of various types and diverse origins. Science, 130:267, 1959.
12. Berlin, L., Goodell, H., and Wolff, H. G.: Relation of pain perception and central inhibitory effect of noxious stimulation to phenomenon of extinction of pain. Arch. Neurol., 80:533, 1958.
13. Best, C. H., and Taylor, H. B.: The Physiological Basis of Medical Practice. ed. 8. Baltimore, Williams and Wilkins, 1966.
14. Billars, K. S.: You have pain? I think this will help. Am. J. Nurs., 70:2143, 1970.
15. Bing, E.: Six Practical Lessons for an Easier Childbirth. New York, Bantam Books, Inc., 1969.
16. Blaylock, J.: The psychological and cultural influences on the reaction to pain: a review of the literature. Nurs. Forum, 7:262, 1968.
17. Bochnak, M. A., Rhymes, J. P., and Leonard, R. C.: The comparison of two types of nursing activity on the relief of pain. Innovations in Nurse-Patient Relationships: Automatic or Reasoned Nurse Actions, Clinical Papers No. 6, p. 5, New York, American Nurses' Association, 1962.
18. Bonner, H.: Group Dynamics: Principles and Applications. p. 14, New York, Ronald Press Co., 1959.

19. Boyd, E. M.: The safety and toxicity of aspirin, Am. J. Nurs., *71*:964, 1971.

20. Bronzo, A., Jr., and Powers, G.: Relationship of anxiety with pain threshold. J. Psychol., *66:*181, 1967.

21. Bruegel, M. A. Relationship of preoperative anxiety to perception of postoperative pain. Nurs. Res., *20*:26, 1971.

22. Cannon, W. B.: Bodily Changes in Pain, Hunger, Fear and Rage. ed. 2. New York, D. Appleton-Century, 1929.

23. Chaffee, E. E., and Greisheimer, E. M.: Basic Physiology and Anatomy. ed. 2. Philadelphia, J. B. Lippincott, 1969.

24. Chambers, W. G., and Price, G. G.: Influence of nurse upon effects of analgesics administered. Nurs. Res., *16*:228, 1967.

25. Chapman, W. P. Measurements of pain sensitivity in normal control subjects and in psychoneurotic subjects. Psychosom. Med., *6*:252, 1944.

26. Chertok, L.: Motherhood and Personality: Psychosomatic Aspects of Childbirth. Philadelphia, Tavistock Publications and J. B. Lippincott, 1969.

27. Clark, J. W., and Bindra, D.: Individual differences in pain thresholds. Canad. J. Psychol., *10*:69, 1956.

28. Collins, L. G.: Pain sensitivity and ratings of childhood experience. Percept. Mot. Skills, *21*:349, 1965.

29. Current Research on Sleep and Dreams. Public Health Service Publication No. 1389, Washington, D.C., U. S. Government Printing Office, 1965.

30. Dickinson, E.: The Mystery of Pain. *In* Love Poems, p. 51. Mount Vernon, Peter Pauper Press, n.d.

31. Dodson, H. C., and Bennett, H. A.: Relief of postoperative pain. Am. Surg., *20:*405, 1954.

32. Eckenhoff, J. E.: The anesthesiologist and the management of pain. J. Chronic Dis., *4:*96, 1956.

33. Elliott, H. C.: Textbook of Neuroanatomy. Philadelphia, J. B. Lippincott, 1969.

34. Engel, B. T.: Some physiological correlates of hunger and pain. J. Exp. Psychol., *57*:389, 1959.

35. Farnsworth, D.: Pain and the individual. New Eng. J. Med., *254*:559, 1956.

36. Festinger, L.: Cognitive dissonance. Sci. Am., *207:*93, 1962.

37. Flavell, J. H.: The Developmental Psychology of Jean Piaget. New York, D. Van Nostrand Co., Inc., 1963.

38. Gliedman, L. H., *et al.*: Some implications of conditioned reflex studies for placebo research. Am. J. Psychiat., *113:*1103, 1957.

39. Gonda, T. A.: Pain and addiction in terminal illness. *In* Schoenberg, B., *et al.* (eds.): Loss and Grief: Psychological Management in Medical Practice. chap. 17, p. 261, New York, Columbia University Press, 1970.

40. Halsell, M.: Moist heat for the relief of postoperative pain. Am. J. Nurs., *67*:767, 1967.

41. Hardy, J. D.: The nature of pain. J. Chronic Dis., *4*:22, 1956.

42. Hardy, J. D., Wolff, H. G., and Goodell, H.: Pain threshold in man. Proc. Assoc. Res. Nerv. Men. Dis., *23*:1, 1943.

43. Hardy, J. D., Wolff, H. G., and Goodell, H.: Pain Sensations and Reactions. Baltimore, Williams and Wilkins, 1952. (a)

44. Hardy, J. D., Wolff, H. G., and Goodell, H.: Pricking pain threshold in different body areas. Proc. Soc. Exp. Biol. Med., *80*:425, 1952. (b)

45. Hare, A. P.: Interpersonal relations in the small group. *In* Faris, R. E. L., (ed.): Handbook of Modern Sociology. chap. 7, p. 217. Chicago, Rand McNally and Co., 1964.

46. Harris, B. L.: Who needs written care plans anyway? Am. J. Nurs., *70*:2136, 1970.

47. Healy, K. M.: Does preoperative instruction make a difference? Am. J. Nurs., *68*:62, 1968.

48. Herrnstein, R. J.: Placebo effect in the rat. Science, *138*:677, 1962.

49. Hill, H. E., Kornetsky, C. H., Flanary, H. G., and Wikler, A.: Studies on anxiety associated with anticipation of pain. Arch. Neurol. Psychiat., *67*:612, 1952.

50. Hodges, W. F.: Effects of ego threat and threat of pain on state anxiety. J. Personality Soc. Psychol., *8*:364, 1968.

51. Hofling, C. K., and Leninger, M. M., and Begg, E.: Basic Psychiatric Concepts in Nursing. Philadelphia, J. B. Lippincott, 1967.

52. Janis, I. L.: Psychological Stress. p. 374. New York, John Wiley and Sons, 1958.

53. Jarvis, D.: Open heart surgery: patients' perceptions of care. Am. J. Nurs., *70*:2591, 1970.

54. Johnson, D. E.: Powerlessness: a significant determinant in patient behavior? J. Nurs. Educ., *6*:39, 1967.

55. Jones, A., Bentler, P. M., and Petry, G.: The reduction of uncertainty concerning future pain. J. Abnorm. Psychol., *71*:87, 1966.

56. Kanfer, F. H., and Goldfoot, D. A.: Self-control and tolerance of noxious stimulation. Psychol. Rep., *18*:79, 1966.

57. Kast, E. C.: The measurement of pain: a new approach to an old problem. J. New Drugs, *2*:344, 1962.

58. Kaufmann, M. A., and Brown, D. E.: Pain wears many faces. Am. J. Nurs., *61*:48, 1961.

59. Keats, A. S.: Postoperative pain: research and treatment. J. Chronic Dis., *4*:72, 1956.

60. Keele, K. D.: The vocabulary of pain. Paper delivered at University of California, Los Angeles, Center for the Health Sciences, May 2, 1966.

61. Kroger, W. S., Steinberg, J., (ed.): Childbirth with Hypnosis. Hollywood, Wilshire Book Co., 1965.

62. Lambert, J. P.: Psychiatric observations on children with abdominal pain. Am. J. Psychiat., *98*:451, 1941-42.

63. Lasagna, L. C.: The clinical measurement of pain. Ann. N.Y. Acad. Sci., *86*:29, 1960.

64. Lasagna, L., Laties, V. G., and Dohan, J. L.: Further studies on the "pharmacology" of placebo administration. J. Clin. Invest., *37*:533, 1958.

65. Lasagna, L., Mosteller, F., von Felsinger, J. M., and Beecher, H. K.: A study of the placebo response. Am. J. Med., *16*:770, 1954.

66. Layton, Sister M. M.: Behavior therapy and its implications for psychiatric nursing. Perspect. Psychiat. Care, *4*:38, 1966.

67. Liberman, R.: An analysis of the placebo phenomenon. J. Chronic Dis., *15*:761, 1962.

68. Lim, R. K. S.: Pain mechanisms. Anesthesiology, *28*:106, 1967.

69. Livingston, W. K.: Pain Mechanisms. New York, Macmillan, 1943.

70. Loan, W. B., and Dundee, J. W.: The clinical assessment of pain. Practitioner, *198*:759, 1967. (a)

71. Loan, W. B., and Dundee, J. W.: The value of postoperative pain in the assessment of analgesics. Brit. J. Anaesth., *39*:743, 1967. (b)
72. Loan, W. B., and Morrison, J. D. The incidence and severity of postoperative pain. Brit. J. Anaesth., *39*:695, 1967.
73. Loewenstein, W. R.: On the "specificity" of a sensory receptor. J. Neurophysiol., *24*:150, 1961.
74. Malmo, R., and Shagass, C.: Physiologic studies to reaction to stress in anxiety and early schizophrenia. Psychosom. Med., *11*:9, 1949.
75. Masson, A. H.: The role of analgesic drugs in the treatment of postoperative pain. Brit. J. Anaesth., *39*:713, 1967.
76. Masuda, M., and Dudley, D. L.: Physiologic responses to noxious head stimuli. J. Psychom. Res., *12*:205, 1968.
77. McBride, M.A. B.: "Pain" and effective nursing practice. Session 5. Scientific Bases for Therapeutic Nursing Practice—Evaluation of Nursing Action, p. 75. American Nurses' Association Clinical Sessions, American Nurses' Association, 1966 in San Francisco. New York, Appleton-Century-Crofts, 1967.
78. MBride, M.A.: The additive to the analgesic. Am. J. Nurs., *69*:974, 1969.
79. McCabe, G. S.: Cultural influences on patient behavior. Am. J. Nurs., *60*:1101, 1960.
80. McCaffery, M.: Nursing Practice Theories Related to Cognition, Bodily Pain, and Man-Environment Interactions. Los Angeles, UCLA Student's Store, 1968.
81. McCaffery, M.: Brief episodes of pain in children. *In* Bergersen, B. S., *et al.*: Current Concepts in Clinical Nursing. vol. II, chap. 17, p. 178. St. Louis, C. V. Mosby, 1969.
82. McCaffery, M., and Moss, F.: Nursing intervention for bodily pain. Am. J. Nurs., *67*:1224, 1967.
83. Melzack, R.: Pain perception. Res. Publ. Ass. Res. Nerv. Ment. Dis., *48*:272, 1970. (a)
84. Melzack, R.: Phantom limbs. Psychol. Today, *4*:63, 1970. (b)
85. Melzack, R., and Scott, T. H.: The effects of early experience on the response to pain. J. Comp. Physiol. Psychol., *50*:155, 1957.
86. Melzack, R., and Wall, P. D.: Pain mechanisms: a new theory. Science, *150*:971, 1965.
87. Melzack, R., and Wall, P. D.: Psychophysiology of pain. International Anesthesiology Clinics, Anesth. Neurophysio., *8*:3, 1970.
88. Melzack, R., Weisz, A. Z., and Sprague, L. T.: Strategems for controlling pain: contributions of auditory stimulation and suggestion. Exper. Neurol., *8*:239, 1963.
89. Mezzanotte, E. J.: Group instruction in preparation for surgery. Am. J. Nurs., *70*:89, 1970.
90. Morgenstern, F. S.: The effects of sensory input and concentration on postamputation phantom limb pain. J. Neurol. Neurosurg. Psychiat., *27*:58, 1964.
91. Moss, F. T., and Meyer, B.: The effects of nursing interaction upon pain relief in patients. Nurs. Res., *15*:303, 1966.
92. Nichols, J. R.: How opiates change behavior. Scientific Am., *212*:80, 1965.
93. Noordenbos, W.: Pain. Amsterdam, Elsevier, 1959.
94. Pain. Med. World News, *11*:26, 1970.
95. Palisin, H. E.: Nursing care plans are a snare and a delusion. Am. J. Nurs., *71*:63, 1971.

96. Pavlov, I. P., Anrep, G. V., (ed. and tr.): Conditioned Reflexes. Oxford, University Press, 1927.

97. Pavlov, I. P.: Lectures on Conditioned Reflexes. New York, International Publishers, 1928.

98. Peck, R. E.: A precise technique for the measurement of pain. Headache, 7:189, 1967.

99. Peters, J., Benjamin, F. B., Helvey, W. M., and Albright, G. A.: Study of sensory deprivation, pain and personality relationships for space travel. NASA TN D-2113. New York, Republic Aviation Corporation for National Aeronautics and Space Administration, Washington, D.C., Sept., 1963.

100. Petrie, A., Collins, W., and Solomon, P.: The tolerance for pain and for sensory deprivation. Am. J. Psychol., 73:80, 1960.

101. Piaget, J.: Judgement and Reasoning in the Child. Totowa, N. J., Littlefield, Adams and Co., 1959.

102. Psychophysical Preparation for Childbearing: Guidelines for Teaching. ed. 2. New York, Maternity Center Association, 1965.

103. Ramzy, I., and Wallerstein, R. S.: Pain, fear and anxiety: a study in their interrelationships. Psychonal. Study Child, 13:147, 1958.

104. Rayport, M.: Addiction problems in the medical use of narcotic analgesics. J. Chronic Dis., 4:102, 1956.

105. Riehl, J. P.: The effect of naturally occurring pain on the galvanic skin response and heart rate: a clinical study. Unpublished masters thesis, University of California at Los Angeles, 1965.

106. Schachter, S.: The Psychology of Affiliation. p. 12. Stanford, Calif., Stanford University Press, 1959.

107. Schamp. J. R., and H. M.: Variability of pain threshold in man. J. Dent. Res., 25:101, 1946.

108. Schultz, D. P.: Sensory Restriction. New York, Academic Press, 1965.

109. Seeman, M., and Evans, J. W.: Alienation and learning in a hospital setting. Am. Sociol., Rev., 27:772, 1962.

110. Selye, H.: The general adaptation syndrome and diseases of adaptation. J. Clin. Endocr., 6:217, 1946.

111. Selye, H.: The Stress of Life. New York, McGraw-Hill, 1956.

112. Shor, R. E.: Physiological effects of painful stimulation during hypnotic analgesia under conditions designed to minimize anxiety. Int. J. Clin. Exp. Hypn., 10:183, 1962.

113. Smith, D. M.: Writing objectives as a nursing practice skill. Am. J. Nurs., 7:319, 1971.

114. Sternbach, R. A.: Principles of Psychophysiology. New York, Academic Press, 1966.

115. Sternbach, R. A.: Pain: A Psychophysiological Analysis. New York, Academic Press, 1968.

116. Sternbach, R. A., and Tursky, B.: Ethnic differences among housewives in psychophysical and skin potential responses to electric shock. Psychophysiology, 1:241, 1965.

117. Sweet, W. H.: Pain. *In* Field, J., Magoun, H. W., and Hall, V. E. (eds.): Handbook of Physiology. vol. 1, sec. 1, chap. XIX, p. 459. Washington, D.C., American Physiological Society, 1959.

118. Szasz, T. S.: Language and Pain. *In* Arieti, S., (ed.): American Handbook of Psychiatry. vol. 1, chap. 49, p. 982. New York, Basic Books, 1959.

119. Tingling, D. C., and Klein, R. F.: Psychogenic pain and aggression: the syndrome of the solitary hunter. Psychosom. Med., 28:738, 1966.

120. Tursky, B., and Sternbach, R. A.: Further physiological correlates of ethnic differences in responses to shock. Psychophysiology, *4*:67, 1967.
121. Uses of Wine in Medical Practice. San Francisco, Wine Advisory Board, 1967.
122. Vaughn, G. F.: Children in hospital. Lancet, *1*:1117, 1957.
123. Walike, B. C., and Meyer, B.: Relation between placebo reactivity and selected personality factors. Nurs. Res., *15*:119, 1966.
124. Watts, A. W.: Pain. *In* Eastern Wisdom and Modern Life. San Francisco, Educational Television and Radio Center, shown June 9, 1969.
125. Webb, C.: Tactics to reduce a child's fear of pain. Am. J. Nurs., *66*:2698, 1966.
126. Weddell, A. G. M.: "Activity pattern" hypothesis for sensation of pain. *In* Grenell, R. G., (ed.): Progress in Neurobiology, vol. V, Neural Physiopathology, p. 134. New York, Paul B. Hoeber, 1962.
127. Whitney, L. R.: Behavioral approaches to the nursing of the mentally retarded. Nurs. Clin. N. Am., *1*:641, 1966. (a)
128. Whitney, L. R.: Operant learning theory: a framework deserving nursing investigation. Nurs. Res., *15*:229, 1966. (b)
129. Winton, F. R., and Bayliss, L. E.: Human Physiology. ed. 5. Boston, Little, Brown and Co., 1962.
130. Wolf, S.: The pharmacology of placebos. Pharmacol. Rev., *11*:689, 1959.
131. Wolff, B. B., and Horland, A. A.: Effect of suggestion upon experimental pain: a validation study. J. Abnorm. Psychol., *72*:402, 1967.
132. Wolff, H. G.: Stress and Disease. Springfield, Ill. Charles C Thomas, 1953.
133. Wolff, H., and Wolf., S.: Pain. ed. 2. Springfield, Ill., Charles C Thomas, 1958.
134. Zaporozhets, A. V.: Development of perception in the preschool age child. Soc. Res. Child Dev. Mono., Chicago, Ill., University of Chicago Press, *30*:82, 1965.
135. Zborowski, M.: Cultural components in responses to pain. J. Soc. Issues, *8*:16, 1952.
136. Zborowski, M.: People in Pain. San Francisco, Jossey-Bass Inc., 1969.
137. Zimbardo, P. G., Cohen, A. R., Weisenberg, M., Dworkin, L., and Firestone, I.: Control of pain motivation by cognitive dissonance. Science, *151*:217, 1966.

Supplementary Bibliography

Barber, T. X.: The effects of "hypnosis" on pain: a critical review of experimental and clinical findings. Psychosom. Med., *25*:303, 1963.
Conway, B.: The seventh right, Am. J. Nurs., *70*:1040, 1970.
Crowley, D. M.: Pain and Its Alleviation. Los Angeles, Regents of the University of California, 1962.
Finneson, B. E.: Diagnosis and Management of Pain Syndrome, Philadelphia, W. B. Saunders, 1967.
Fischer, H. K.: The problem of pain from the psychiatrist's viewpoint. Psychosomatics, *9*:319, 1968.
Keele, K. D.: The pain chart. Lancet, *2*:3, 1948.
Knighton, R.: Pain. Boston, Little, Brown and Co., 1966.
LeShan, L.: The world of the patient in severe pain of long duration. J. Chronic Dis., *17*:337, 1964.

MacBryde, C. M. (ed.): Signs and Symptoms. ed. 5, chaps. 3, 4, 5, 6, 7, 8, 9, 10, 11, 12 and 13. Philadelphia, J. B. Lippincott, 1970.

McBride, M. A. B.: Nursing approach, pain, and relief: an exploratory experiment. Nurs. Res., *16*:337, 1967.

McKee, K.: Neurotic bodily pain in children. Am. J. Nurs., *70*:130, 1970.

Merskey, H., and Spear, F. G.: Pain: Psychological and Psychiatric Aspects. London, Bailliere, Tindall and Cassell, 1967.

Pain, Part 1, Basic Concepts and Assessment. Am. J. Nurs., *66*:1085, 1966.

Pain, Part 2, Rationale for Intervention. Am. J. Nurs., *66*:1345, 1966.

Seaman, B.: Man Against Pain. Philadelphia, Chilton Co., 1962.

Smith, M. M.: Nursing knowledge and activity in relation to the period of anticipation of pain in the adult. *In* Solving "Difficult" Problems in Nursing Care, Clinical papers no. 20, p. 25. New York, American Nurses' Association, 1962.

Therrien, B., and Salmon, J. H.: Percutaneous cordotomy for relief of intractable pain. Am. J. Nurs., *68*:2594, 1968.

Way, E. L. (ed.): New Concepts in Pain and Its Clinical Management. Philadelphia, F. A. Davis, 1967.

Index

Numerals in **boldface** indicate a figure.
A "t" following a page number indicates a table concerning the subject mentioned.